Acclaim for *The Professional Yoga Teacher's Handbook*

. . . .

"This incredibly useful handbook covers every facet of yoga teaching, from landing your first teaching job to refining your yoga-teaching language. Whether you're an aspiring yoga teacher or have years of experience behind you, this guide will help you level-up your teaching craft and career within the current landscape of the modern yoga world."—**Jenni Rawlings,** pioneer of science-based yoga, movement, and instruction

"Dr. Rountree incorporates her wide-ranging experience as a dedicated yogi, author, business owner, athlete, and master teacher to enhance and support the careers of yoga instructors at any stage of their professional journey. She offers advice with a practical workbook that allows the reader to ask thoughtful, self-reflective questions. An invaluable addition to any yoga teacher's library."—**Ingrid Yang, MD, JD, E-RYT 500, C-IAYT,** author of *Hatha Yoga Asanas* and *Adaptive Yoga*

"No one can predict how the pandemic will continue to impact local yoga communities and the yoga industry at large. Yet Rountree's book is the business-of-yoga book that every 200-hour training program needs to have as required reading. Clear, practical, well-informed, and an honest 'peek behind the curtain' of being a yoga professional, this book is a game changer for yoga teachers who want to teach in an impactful, purposed, and far-reaching way."
—**Octavia Raheem,** co-owner of Sacred Chill West, author of Gather, and yoga teacher

"How I wish I had this book when I first began teaching! Asana knowledge and yogic philosophy will only get you so far. This book points the way to the 'next level' of your aspiration to teach, walking you through a truly integral strategy for the business of teaching yoga. A teacher training without this book is like buying a new car but failing to fill up the tank."
—**Josh Summers,** Yin Yoga trainer and host of the podcast *Everyday Sublime*

"Whether you're embarking on your first teacher training program or you've been teaching for a decade, this book strikes every essential chord while providing a dose of 'real talk.' Relevant to today's yoga culture, this book is an indispensable companion for anyone on the path of teaching yoga."—**Terry Cockburn,** owner and director, Freeport Yoga Company

"*The Professional Yoga Teachers Handbook* is an excellent guide to teaching yoga successfully. It includes sage advice on offering the best quality instruction in today's climate, while setting up healthy boundaries to enjoy the rest of your life."—**Michael Johnson,** founder, Clearlight Yoga

Also by Sage Rountree

The Athlete's Guide to Yoga
The Athlete's Pocket Guide to Yoga
The Athlete's Guide to Recovery
The Runner's Guide to Yoga
Racing Wisely
Everyday Yoga

with Alexandra DeSiato

Lifelong Yoga
Teaching Yoga Beyond the Poses

THE PROFESSIONAL YOGA TEACHER'S HANDBOOK

The Ultimate Guide for Current and Aspiring Instructors

SAGE ROUNTREE

THE EXPERIMENT

NEW YORK

THE PROFESSIONAL YOGA TEACHER'S HANDBOOK: *The Ultimate Guide for Current and Aspiring Instructors*
Copyright © 2020 by Sage Rountree

The Experiment, LLC | 220 East 23rd Street, Suite 600 | New York, NY 10010-4658
theexperimentpublishing.com

This book contains the opinions and ideas of its author. It is intended to provide helpful and informative material on the subjects addressed in the book. It is sold with the understanding that the author and publisher are not engaged in rendering medical, health, or any other kind of personal professional services in the book. The author and publisher specifically disclaim all responsibility for any liability, loss, or risk— personal or otherwise—that is incurred as a consequence, directly or indirectly, of the use and application of any of the contents of this book.

The Experiment's books are available at special discounts when purchased in bulk for premiums and sales promotions as well as for fund-raising or educational use. For details, contact us at info@theexperimentpublishing.com.

Library of Congress Cataloging-in-Publication Data

Names: Rountree, Sage Hamilton, author.
Title: The professional yoga teacher's handbook : the ultimate guide for
   current and aspiring instructors / Sage Rountree.
Description: New York : The Experiment, [2020] | Includes index.
Identifiers: LCCN 2020024420 (print) | LCCN 2020024421 (ebook) | ISBN
   9781615196975 (trade paperback) | ISBN 9781615196982 (ebook)
Subjects: LCSH: Hatha yoga--Study and teaching.
Classification: LCC RA781.7 .R697 2020 (print) | LCC RA781.7 (ebook) |
   DDC 613.7/046--dc23
LC record available at https://lccn.loc.gov/2020024420
LC ebook record available at https://lccn.loc.gov/2020024421

ISBN 978-1-61519-697-5
Ebook ISBN 978-1-61519-698-2

Cover and text design by Jordan Wannemacher | Author photograph by Amelia Cassar

Manufactured in China

First printing September 2020
10 9 8 7 6 5 4 3 2 1

For Martha Harbison

Contents

Preface

· ·

I HATED THE FIRST YOGA CLASS I attended. It was harder than I expected, there were manual corrections and confusing Sanskrit, and savasana was bizarre to me, especially because I desperately had to pee but, unsure of the protocol or how long we'd be lying still, was afraid to leave the room. If I'd felt neutral instead of negative about the experience, you wouldn't be holding this book. My intense aversion led me to go back for more, to get at the root of what made yoga challenging and to see whether I could change my reaction. As I dug deeper into yoga, I garnered the tools to investigate my early response to the practice.

Prenatal yoga was a bridge for me. During my first pregnancy, I found that I was more open to the sense of connection and union that yoga offers, and I was eager to watch what changed in my body and mind moment to moment. Then, during my second pregnancy, I felt the call to be a yoga teacher. Every class I've taken—especially that first one—has shown me something new about the practice and taught me how to be the best version of myself, both as a practitioner and as a student.

Looking back, I can see that my previous experiences had also set me up to be a yoga teacher. Both my parents are educators, and I didn't stray far from the cozy nest of academia, going straight from college to graduate school, where I eventually earned a PhD in English literature. During graduate school, I came to running as a stress release, and my running led me back to yoga for good. After graduation, I realized that I could use the skills I'd learned in graduate school in the yoga field. I'd spent my educational career learning how to teach, how to help my peers grow as teachers, and how to research the subjects that interested me, like the intersection between sports and yoga. Eventually, I was able to use my experience writing to share my research with readers. This is my ninth book.

I entered yoga teacher training in 2003. Though I'd only been out of the classroom for a few years, it was wonderful to get back into concerted study. Teacher training gives you a chance to explore things you won't get in a regular class and to pursue your special interests. In teacher training, we have a special opportunity to form friendships in a group of like-minded people. This is how we spent our childhoods and young adulthoods—studying alongside classmates—and it feels like coming home to get back to it. If you haven't already taken teacher training, I know this communion—having colleagues who are interested in the same things that you're passionate about, and growing together—will be a special part of your experience.

The more I practice yoga, the more I depend on the simplicity of the basics: breath, awareness, easy movement. The same goes for teaching. Coming back to the basics will keep you professional. I am still learning in every class. I pick up a new use for a prop, admire a new turn of phrase, or hear an old lesson imparted in a way that gives it new relevance. Whether you are new to the practice or have decades of experience, if you are an aspiring teacher or have been doing it for years, I hope this book will be useful. Much of what we cover is basic. But being a professional is about covering the basics: establishing clear communication, following through on what you promise, and holding yourself to high standards.

Introduction

· ·

YOGA TEACHER TRAININGS have proliferated in America and around the world in the last decade, with only nominal oversight and inconsistent standards from one to the next. If you're going to spend thousands of dollars and lots of your energy on a teacher training, you probably want to be sure it's worth your time and money. This laxity of oversight may soon change with the imposition of new standards for the Yoga Alliance, but many trainings don't operate under this umbrella, some for good reason and while maintaining their own high standards.

Many teachers graduate with little or no understanding of the true state of the profession—what people are paid, how studios are run, how to manage student behavior—or how to find their first teaching job and to do it well. *The Professional Yoga Teacher's Handbook* will guide you to the highest level of professionalism, benefiting students, teachers, and studios alike. If you are in the early stages of your career or feeling like it's time to get back to basics or learn a new approach, I'll walk you through finding a good fit in a teacher training and what questions to ask as you consider enrolling.

Perhaps you've already done one or more trainings but still have many questions about your teaching. In my work with teachers at all levels, from day one teacher trainees to those with decades of experience, I hear the same concerns: How can I best help my students? How can I keep my teaching fresh? How can I make smart choices about my schedule, my money, and my next steps in this career?

Or maybe you don't want to be a yoga teacher, but instead aim to or already do teach Pilates, Gyrokinesis, Barre, or some other movement modality. You'll still get lots from this book! Since our focus is on the container of your career and class rather than prescribing any particular contents, you'll be able to apply what we cover to your work both immediately and in the long term in various in-person and online settings.

Part 1 takes a look at the big picture. We look at the scope of yoga as it is practiced in the West today, so that you can begin to see how your work as a teacher fits into the landscape. Then I'll challenge you to chart a course and set goals for your service to students, so that you can create reasonable expectations and devise clear next steps to grow as a teacher.

Part 2 narrows the focus to you and your career, offering steps from getting your first job to managing your schedule, money, and energy. Along the way, I'll offer both the studio owner's and studio manager's views on how you can be a positive addition to any studio and every yoga community, as well as the best practices I've developed and witnessed from my decades of teaching.

In part 3, we drill down even more, to look at the individual class. We start by thinking through what you need to do outside the classroom to ensure that each class is a good one. Then we investigate how the choices you make in the room itself, or in producing video, affect student experience. You'll learn ways to improve your teaching after every class, so that the next one is even better.

In part 4, we go even further, exploring ways that you might grow toward your goal, whether it is becoming a full-time teacher, creating online content, owning a studio, developing and leading yoga teacher trainings—or all of the above. We finish with a timeline to keep you on track as you work on your career daily, weekly, monthly, annually, and across the years.

As you see, this book is less a what-to-teach manual than a how-to-teach handbook. If you're interested in just what to teach in any given class, I have several resources for you.

For content—poses and sequences to teach in class—please see my books *The Athlete's Pocket Guide to Yoga*, *Everyday Yoga*, and *Lifelong Yoga*, this last one cowritten with Alexandra DeSiato. For my take on alignment, please see *The Athlete's Guide to Yoga* and *The Runner's Guide to Yoga*, but most of all, please develop and trust your own experience with each asana in your body and those of your students. The best way to learn to teach the poses is to take a wide range of classes from different teachers with a variety of backgrounds, then to practice teaching them to a very broad range of people, paying very close attention to your students.

Complement this survey by reading extensively. One of my favorite yoga books is *Yoga Anatomy* by Leslie Kaminoff and Amy Matthews, which you are likely to pick up first for the gorgeous illustrations but which offers a profound and easily digestible discussion of the concepts of effort and ease in relation to the breath and the cell. Erich Schiffmann's *Yoga: The Spirit and Practice of Moving into Stillness* similarly posits a clear view of the principles and practice of yoga in a way that's easy to understand immediately yet still feels rich when you return to it after years of practice. Donna Farhi's *Teaching Yoga* is a clearly written exploration of the ethics of the teacher-student relationship; read it as a complement to chapter 9 of this book. Then, for deeper information on how to find your voice as a yoga teacher and for how to incorporate themes in your classes, please see my *Teaching Yoga Beyond the Poses*, cowritten with Alexandra DeSiato.

Instead of telling you what to teach, this book will guide you to your own answers by prompting you to ask what your students need to learn. It will help you figure out the best way to present what your students need to know, in a manner that will be easy on you while giving them exactly what they need from you, week in and week out.

As you discover your own answers, you'll find numerous prompts to encourage you to articulate your principles, vision, and plans. These reflections can be handwritten in your teaching journal or typed into a document or your notes program. Please do whatever feels most natural, whatever best suits your learning and teaching styles. Visit yogateacherhandbook.com to download a companion document that collects all the prompts together. You can also connect with me there and let me know how you are growing. I look forward to hearing from you!

PART 1

Charting Your Course

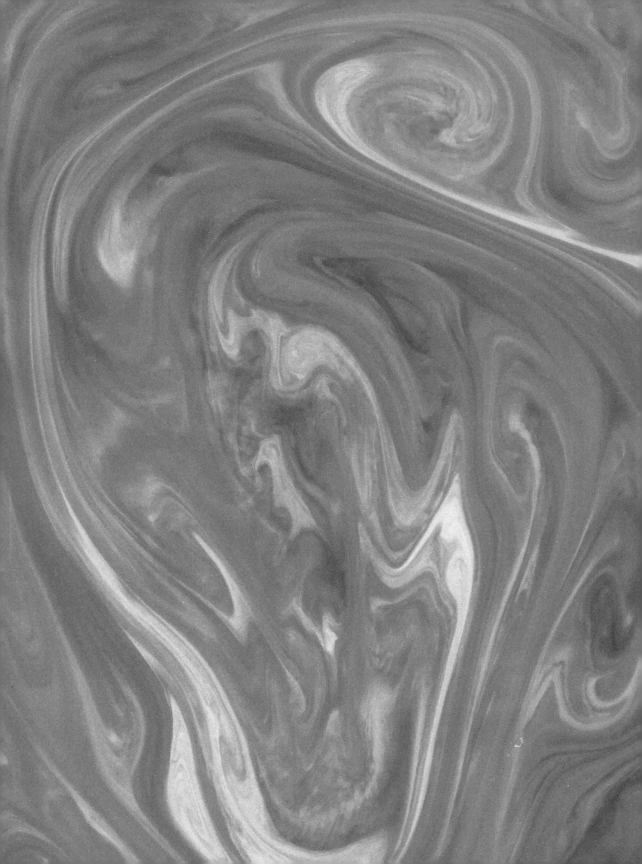

1

So You Want to Be
a Yoga Teacher

. . . .

YOGA HAS HELPED YOU, and now you want to share what you've learned. You've seen your teachers over the years as wise guides and role models, and while you're naturally nervous that you won't be able to fill their shoes, you're starting to feel the urge to try. Great!

Or maybe you've been teaching for a while, but you feel unsure about how to get a studio job, develop a workshop, establish clear boundaries with your students, create online content, or level up in your career. You may simply want to get back to the basics of good teaching. Also great!

Wherever you are in your career, it's useful to step back to see the big picture, check in with your own abilities and goals, and choose a wise path toward where you want to be. These days, there are images of yoga practitioners and teachers coming at you from all angles, and it can be confusing to sift through the chatter to get at the heart of what yoga means to you and then at the question of how you might be able to help others through yoga. Let's start by cutting through the noise.

Look Back on Your Path

Spend some time considering your answers to these questions, then open your journal or a notes file and write about them. You'll find all the workbook prompts in this book at yogateacherhandbook.com.

▶ What led you to yoga?

▶ What do you love about yoga? What does yoga have to teach you? What do you have to teach others about yoga?

▶ What do you find confusing, or off-putting, or difficult about yoga? How can you make peace with these parts of the practice?

▶ Why did you pick up this book? What do you want to learn?

ANYONE IS A POTENTIAL TEACHER

Our teacher trainees at the studio I co-own, Carolina Yoga Company, have included an ex–professional poker player, a current professional salsa dancer, bartenders, grad students, home-schooled sixteen-year-olds, doctors, nurses, lawyers, schoolteachers, stay-at-home moms, and retirees. Anyone can be a yoga teacher. And although being a *good* yoga teacher takes practice, there is nothing that inherently disqualifies you from trying.

The things that make you different from the idealized yoga teacher in your mind's eye (based on what you see in advertising and on your Instagram feed) are the very things that will make you unique and appealing to your students. Recognize what you are bringing to the table. If you have a background in gymnastics and facility with the showier poses, great! This may be your niche. If you have a history as a couch potato, or are rehabbing an injury, great! This can lead to a different niche. Your life experiences will make you sympathetic to the students you can help best. You're best at being exactly who you are. And your authenticity in your personality and your experiences will be the strongest part of your teaching.

Don't let body image stop you from stepping into the seat of the teacher. You do not have to be Instagram-fitfluencer thin and young. There's no shortage of slim, white, economically privileged yoga teachers in the world—and if this is you, you are certainly welcome, too. But what the world really needs is more authentically real people as teachers. The pain points you've discovered in your yoga practice are the very topics on which you'll be the strongest teacher.

And on the other hand, the things that come easiest to you in your practice, whether they be advanced asanas, or relaxing immediately in restorative poses, or sustaining meditation with little effort, will be your biggest blind spots as a teacher. The struggle you have gone through to master whatever is most difficult for you will better equip you to be a helpful teacher. You'll have the experience, the language, and the skills to help others who arrive on their mats looking for guidance just as you once did.

Check Your Blind Spots

Journal on your answers to these questions.

- ▶ What comes easy to you in asana? Are there categories of poses or styles of yoga that you excel at? Why? Is it something in your body, or your mind, or your background? What comes easy to you in breathing, meditation, and the other yoga techniques beyond asana?

- ▶ What do you find challenging? Why is that? Can you drill down on the nature of the challenge?

- ▶ How could these point you toward approaches you should study more? How can recognizing your blind spots help you shore them up?

You Aren't Bryan

I was fortunate to receive some really helpful feedback—some of the most useful teaching advice I've ever heard—after my second public class. I hadn't meant to be teaching that night, and in fact I'd given my first-ever class the evening before. But when the front desk staff told me that the regular teacher, Bryan, wouldn't make it, I eagerly threw my hand in the air and said, "I'll teach the class!" In class, I repeated the sequence I'd prepped for the previous evening, complete with numerous apologies for not teaching the same poses in the same way as Bryan, and while I was nervous, I thought it went pretty well.

The next day, I saw two of the students who'd been in the room. Approaching me, they explained that they were schoolteachers and as such were used to giving and receiving peer critiques. Was I open to hearing some advice? Of course, I said.

"We could tell you weren't Bryan, so you didn't need to apologize for not *being* Bryan," they offered.

What an important thing to be told so early on! Not only did I make the mistake of drawing attention to my self-perceived flaws, I was unnecessarily comparing myself to the regular teacher, which hobbled my own attempt at teaching authentically. It was obvious to the room that I was a different teacher; I didn't need to compare myself or point out all the ways I wasn't him. Instead, I was free to be Sage, authentically and without apology. The students were grateful to have a teacher that evening, rather than no teacher at all.

Remind yourself: You don't have to be Bryan. You don't have to be Sage—only I do. You only have to be yourself.

This experience also taught me to be receptive to student feedback. Don't expect to follow it all, but listen to what your students tell you, as they will be some of your greatest teachers.

THE PERFECT SIDE HUSTLE

Let me be perfectly clear right up front: Teaching yoga is not an ideal primary profession, despite what social media might imply. The market is ever more saturated with teachers; studios are paying less and per hour (we'll discuss the nitty-gritty of money in chapter 5); venues for teaching workshops are on the decline; the big-name yoga festivals don't pay much to presenters. There are only so many hours in a week that you can be physically present to teach. And then, along comes a pandemic to shut down in-person classes!

But while it's not usually the best choice for a full-time job, teaching yoga is a lovely second job. Teaching yoga is my second or third job, after business ownership and writing. At Carolina Yoga Company, we have only a handful of teachers on our large staff across three studios whose sole job is teaching yoga. Far more common is to work a part-time or full-time job in another field, with yoga as a side hustle. Our teachers have all sorts of jobs: working at IBM, running an accounting firm, working for the federal government, and teaching from preschool to college, among others. Those who teach full time are often cushioned by having a partner with a well-paying job. That's certainly the case for me. I recognize this immense privilege, and I strive to use it in the service of helping others.

All the good reasons someone might want to become a yoga teacher have service at their core. The bad reasons have ego: wanting power over others, more rigid control over your own body, or oodles of money. But as the yoga sutras tell us, attachment to ego (*asmita*) causes suffering. Remember that service is at the core of your work. But that doesn't mean that you need to do it for free! The more you are paid for your teaching, the more you'll be able to give your teaching away to those who wouldn't otherwise receive it.

As you work through the prompts in this book, consider how you can best serve yourself and others on your yoga journey. This might mean finding ways to bring yoga to underserved populations, especially groups that would never think of yoga as a help for them or would never make it in to a studio. Later, we'll explore how you might eventually grow a part-time job as a yoga teacher into your full-time profession. But now, let's talk about how to get started.

Have Clear Eyes about Teacher Training

For many, teacher training is the first step to becoming a yoga teacher. Whether you are considering your first teacher training, continuing in an advanced-studies program, or developing a specialty, it's useful to do some math to see what's feasible. List here:

▶ The price(s) of the training(s) you are considering. If there's more than one, compare their rates.

▶ How much money and time you have available or will need to budget to cover the costs, factoring in any income you'd lose from not being available to work your regular job or teach your regular classes during your training.

▶ How long you will need to work to earn back what you have spent. If you're savvy, do this in a spreadsheet. At the lower end of the spectrum, factor earning $20/teaching hour (not including travel or planning time) coming out of teacher training. At the upper end, plug in $60. And if you know for sure that finishing an advanced training would guarantee you more than that, or if you're already teaching private lessons at higher rates, add these to your projections.

Given the above, is yoga teacher training (YTT) the best next step for you, or would doing an intensive to deepen your knowledge without being on a teacher track be smarter? You could also consider joining a work-study program. Some studios also offer a discount on trainings for people who've been working there for some time. Make notes on the next steps based on your responses.

TEACHING YOUR FIRST CLASSES

If you take part in teacher training, your first class will usually happen in that context. Trainees may be encouraged to create their own small classes for family and friends, or to take yoga into the community. During the Carolina Yoga Company teacher training and immediately after, trainees are invited to cut their teeth in our community class, which is $5 to students and unpaid for teachers. We equate it to getting your hair cut at the beauty school—students get a low rate in exchange for helping the teachers practice and grow. The studio provides the students, so all trainees need to do is show up and teach. It's a wonderful first step toward teaching in a studio setting, with props, dimmable lighting, support for music, and all the amenities. Many studios have such programs; if yours does not, consider suggesting it to the owner and/or manager.

The obvious next step after teacher training is to start teaching somewhere you are needed. This can be a community group, a gym, a yoga-in-the-park offering, in a special-interest group online—anywhere that lets you continue to practice and grow. This could be paid work or volunteer work. It's also a wonderful ongoing practice, especially if you've been teaching for a while and feel like your teaching is getting stale. Taking your work out of the studio setting and into the community helps bring yoga's gifts to those who need it most, while also reigniting your passion for the practice.

You might also consider a work-study program to get your foot in the door. At Carolina Yoga Company, several of our graduates are on our teaching roster. Most of them came through our work-study program, which gets new staff up to speed on our procedures and keeps potential new teachers top of mind when we write our quarterly teaching schedule. Many studios have such a program; if not, consider suggesting one or working the front desk. Being a work-study student is like joining the farm team; moving to the sub list is like getting to AAA baseball. You might get called up in a pinch, so performing well and being easy to work with can earn you a spot on the major-league roster. All along the way, you're getting an inside view of the organization, its systems, and its values.

A MENTORSHIP

One of the best ways to grow in yoga, both as a student and as a teacher, is to seek and nurture a healthy relationship with a mentor. Even though the typical class features only one teacher, no one teaches in a vacuum. Every teacher has a support staff of her own mentors, peers, manager, and classmates (because continuing to be a student is critical). Knowing who yours are early on will ensure you have the strength of your team throughout your career. When you find a teacher who lights you up, whether it's in a regular class, in a continuing education training, or online, introduce yourself. If the time is right, ask about their background and path. You might find ideas in this teacher's experience to guide you on your journey. Ask respectfully whether they have the time to help you in the future, and if so, how they prefer you contact them.

A healthy mentorship will leave you feeling both supported and appropriately challenged to grow. A good mentor will point out opportunities for you—workshops you might take or teach, books you should read, skills you should hone. They can also open doors for you, by making introductions to host venues, book agents, private clients, and so on.

Being a mentor is also deeply rewarding. When you have successfully navigated some portion of the field, look for newer teachers whom you can mentor through this experience. You don't need to have been in the field for long to have a lot to offer. In fact, when you are still relatively new, your experience and your takeaways are most fresh. Share them by looking for someone who can benefit from your help, then give it liberally.

Find Your Team

Identify your yoga role models, who can serve as cheerleaders and mentors on your support team as your career grows. Your team could include a teacher you practice with weekly, a family member who has been studying for a long time, or even a friend who first brought you to the practice. Make a list of these team-mates, talk to them about your calling to teach or your inspiration to further develop your career, and chat together about where they see your strengths and suggested next steps.

I'm honored to be on your team, even if we never interact one-on-one. I hope this book will give you all the advice you need from me. If you think of further questions for me, please send them using the email link at yogateacherhandbook.com. I'll do my best to respond and, when my answer has broader application, I'll share it at the site and on my social media (@sagerountree).

2

Education and
Personal Development

· ·

YOGA IS AN EXTREMELY BROAD TERM that covers many practices, from *bhakti* and *japa yoga* (prayer and mantra repetition) to *karma yoga* (selfless service) to *hatha yoga* (finding connection through yoga poses). With the acceptance of yoga in Western culture in the twentieth century came codification of different styles of hatha yoga. As these styles have crystallized, they have become recognizable brands with clear rules about how things are done. You could choose a training in Ashtanga Yoga, with set sequences to progress through. Or you could be studying Sivananda Yoga, or Baptiste Yoga—maybe even directly from Baron Baptiste—or Core Power Yoga, or Insert Any Name Here Yoga. In this chapter, we'll explore how you can find the right path for you to start on, continue on, or change course toward, and how you can then pursue study, both in the context of yoga teacher training and in your own self-study, to deepen your understanding of yoga and your ability to serve others through teaching.

LINEAGES

For context, consider dog breeding. (Bear with me!) Pedigreed dogs are bred to display a particular mix of physical attributes, service skills, and temperament. Done well, this breeding leads to a recognizable brand with discrete abilities. When you buy or adopt a German Shorthaired Pointer, for example, you can expect an athletic dog with high energy, sensitivity to birds, and a brown-and-white spotted shorthair coat. When you buy or adopt a pug, you're expecting something different! Pedigree yields strengths—knowing what you're getting—but it also brings weaknesses. For example, overbreeding can lead to all kinds of health issues, from breathing problems to hip dysplasia. Unscrupulous breeders can mistreat their animals and scam their customers.

On the other hand, nature yields many hybrid dogs. We affectionately call them mutts. These mixed-breed dogs can be stronger overall, as they draw from a broader gene pool and can thus pull strengths from the bloodlines of both parents. Then again, sometimes mutts can have a strange combination of temperament and size, or the legs of a short dog but the body of a long dog (we had one of these as a pet!), which can create structural problems with age.

As we see, there are strengths and weaknesses in both purebred and mixed-breed dogs. Similarly, there are strengths and weaknesses in being attached to one, and only one, lineage, and there are strengths and weaknesses in choosing to draw from many.

If you cast your lot with one particular style, you can expect clear rules about what is in the tradition and what is not, what is canon, and what is not. This can be deeply comforting, as there is usually a right way to do things—poses, meditations, breath exercises, even choosing your wardrobe—and a wrong way. Once you are clear on the right way, you can strive to do things right, and you'll be able to measure your progress along the way. But this has a shadow side, in that such clear-cut traditions often amass power in the hands of a single charismatic leader or cabal of senior teachers or practitioners, and such power can then be abused. For more on the dynamics of high-demand groups and the history of abuse in yoga, see Matthew Remski's book *Practice and All Is Coming: Abuse, Cult Dynamics, and Healing in Yoga and Beyond*. In addition, subscribing to a single dogma excludes other approaches that might help both you and your students. Be careful that service to the fundamentals of a style does not become rigid fundamentalism.

Many of the styles of yoga that are spelled with capital letters—Ashtanga Yoga, Iyengar Yoga, Sivananda Yoga, Anusara Yoga—subscribe to a set of clearly delineated rules, and sometimes their physical practices follow clearly delineated sequences. In Ashtanga Yoga, for example, there are series of prescribed postures that each practitioner learns in order, beginning with the Primary Series. In Bikram Yoga, teachers lead the same twenty-six poses and two breath exercises using the same language (a memorized script of Bikram Choudhury leading the practice, grammatical quirks and all) every single time.

When you take a teacher training in a particular lineage, you'll go deep rather than broad. You can expect to learn the key elements of the lineage, and you might be directed to more and more trainings at further levels to deepen your understanding. It's like doing the Red Cross swim lessons: There's a clear curriculum for each level, and you'll be tested on the skills taught to pass one level and move to the next. Remember: You can also learn to swim in non–Red Cross programs, and some people learn to swim from their friends and family instead of a regulated program. To return to the dog-breeding analogy, in some of these lineages—Iyengar Yoga, for example—you'll be tested on your ability to show the examiners just what they want to see. It's a little like the judges at a dog show: They are looking for certain qualities representative of a breed. Not meeting them doesn't mean the dog is a bad dog!

Research Lineages

While it's useful to know the major lineages of yoga, they aren't relevant to your personal development and teacher training if you can't find a teacher or studio to study with. Thus you'll either need access to these resources nearby or the money and time to travel for them.

Take a look at the offerings in your area, or in places you might reasonably visit. Look at the titles used to describe the classes and approaches. When you see a proper noun, do some research on the style. Look not only at the studio site and the style's webpage but also the search results, to see if there's a history of abuse or impropriety associated with the style. Unfortunately, this is all too common. If you discover that a certain style has a distasteful history, do more research and explore others that align better with your ethics. For styles that interest you, research potential classes you can take; list them and create a plan to visit them.

RESPONSIBLE ECLECTICISM

At Carolina Yoga Company, we embrace what we call "responsible eclecticism." That means we value many different styles, as well as hybrid styles, and we believe the most balanced practice, and therefore the most useful one, involves moving beyond one single approach to include whatever best suits the student day to day, season to season.

Similarly, our yoga teacher training is responsibly eclectic. We go broad. We take our teacher trainees on a tour of the main styles of yoga practiced in America today, while keeping our eyes open about the potential downsides of clinging to one and only one approach. We bring in guest presenters who can speak with authority about the various styles of yoga, because they specialize. (We call this a "great books" approach, in which we go directly to the primary text, as it were.) Put together, these teachers generate a rich tapestry that includes an overview of the various paths up the mountain of yoga. As a result of this broad exposure, our teacher trainees emerge not as cookie-cutter instructors ready to teach the one sequence or the one style they learned but as unique teachers ready to serve their students in whatever way will work best.

If you choose a training that goes deep rather than broad, you may supplement it by taking field trips of your own design. Seek out teachers who offer styles different from what you were exposed to in your training. Research the style in advance: read about it online, watch videos of the style, learn about its key principles and teachers. If the situation allows, ask your teacher how they came to this style and what they find most helpful. This is a useful ongoing practice no matter how long you've been teaching. If you haven't had an experience with hot yoga, aerial yoga, yoga nidra, yoga with weights, Buti Yoga, or whatever is popular in your area, go with an open mind and heart.

Supplement your primary teacher training by voraciously taking classes in a wide range of styles. This is one of the best ways to serve your own students. Knowing what's out there in the wide world of yoga will help you when you have students whose background is limited to a particular style. You'll be able to quickly explain the difference between their previous experience and what will happen in your class—that is, you'll be able to manage student expectations so that you can then fulfill these expectations as you teach.

For example, if at the start of your flow class you meet a new student who's had only hot yoga classes, you might say, "Super! A couple of things to consider: First, obviously, the room is not warm. Pay special attention to how the poses feel different, and don't push the first round of any movement too far. We'll spend ten minutes low to the ground, forty minutes moving, then we'll come back down to the mat for slow unwinding. In that moving segment, there will be a decent amount of upper-body work, so please listen to your wrists, elbows, and shoulders, and feel free to hold plank or to take child's pose instead of what you'll hear me call out as *vinyasa*. We will finish with a led *savasana* of about eight minutes—I'll guide you into it, then sit quietly before talking you out. I'll check in after class and look forward to hearing about how the new experience felt!"

Since in many hot styles there is no vinyasa of *chaturanga*-up dog–down dog, this alerts the student to what's coming and encourages self-care. Some schools of hot yoga end with the students encouraged to take savasana (and it's pronounced differently, to boot, with an initial *s* instead of *sh* sound) for as long as they like, but the teacher leaves the room as they begin their rest. Students who are used to these protocols are going to be surprised to see how things go in the flow class. These few lines of explanation offer a road map so that your students can have a more satisfying experience.

PRODUCTIVE CONFUSION AND CHANGE OVER TIME

If the beauty of subscribing to a particular lineage is clarity, the beauty—and the frustration—of being responsibly eclectic is running up against contradictions. You might, at the very same studio on the very same day, be taught triangle pose in two very different ways, each illuminating and useful. Teachers can make very persuasive arguments for why you might do a pose their way—it can be based on lineage, or their understanding of anatomy, or their own workarounds in coping with injuries. How can you then tell the right way to do triangle pose?

We'll explore in the next chapter whether there is a right way to do yoga. When your previous understanding of the "right" way to do things butts up against a new approach, you're put in a productive state of confusion. The way to resolve it is through practice and continued study. Talk to the teachers who offer conflicting approaches, and get to know how and why they have reached their conclusions. As you find yourself in states of dissonance, you have a chance to practice equanimity, finding center even in the face of shifting circumstance. This is an important skill for everyone, and especially for yoga teachers. The more you study and grow your knowledge, the more you'll see how much you don't know, and you'll find ways to make peace with that.

As you continue to practice, study, and teach yoga, and especially as your body changes with age, you'll necessarily hit pain points where your previous experience and beliefs no longer seem to apply. These are useful for self-study, and they may eventually prompt you to adapt your practice within a particular style or to cast your net wider. You may find yourself drawn to practicing or teaching yoga nidra, or yin yoga, or restorative yoga—or, conversely, to finding complementary practices like Pilates that balance your flexibility-focused yoga practice with strength-based exercise.

These moments of productive confusion are teachers. They may be what led you to pick up this book, and they should be what leads you to deeper study. This could be taking a yoga teacher training, further study in your current style or school, or a jump to a different approach as you seek to find new truths.

TEACHER TRAINING STANDARDS

The Yoga Alliance (YA) Registered Yoga School (RYS) system is an attempt to guarantee a consistently high quality of teacher education—a noble and useful goal. It's only one system, though, and you can still be a wonderful teacher without ever attending a formal yoga teacher training—or if you take one outside of the YA world. By the same token, graduating from a YA-registered school is no guarantee of a good teacher. Learning about the YA's structure and its standards can help you make an informed choice about whether you will buy in.

The YA is a registry. That means that teachers pay to have their names added to the YA's rolls and to use its registered symbols. It's not a certifying body or a regulatory one, and it's not designed to enforce any yoga rules. Instead, it sets standards of its own, and teachers and schools can align with them and pay to be registered.

As a teacher, you are *certified* by your school, and then you may choose to *register* with the YA. In order to keep your registration current, you are required to self-report the continuing education you have undergone (and, of course, pay another fee). Naturally, I encourage lots of continuing education, over and above the YA standards and whether you are inside the YA universe or not, because learning is a lifelong process and yoga is a living, changing system.

Ultimately, you will decide whether registering with the Yoga Alliance is right for you (more on this later). As you make your decision, remember this: Your students want to feel better after your class. They don't care whether you hold a 200- or 500- or even a 1,000-hour certification. Your *employers* may care, especially if you are teaching at a gym, where management that doesn't come from a yoga background will want to know you're held to a national standard. At some studios, your pay rate will depend directly on how much yoga education you've had. Read on for more info on each of the certifications.

200 Hours

Most trainings in the West target the 200-hour model and the Yoga Alliance standards. Internationally, you will find different models, both shorter and longer. And there are some systems, such as YogaFit, that run shorter weekend trainings, often geared toward fitness professionals with previous group exercise experience. Somewhat confusingly, 200-hour trainings are not required to have 200 classroom hours—the Yoga Alliance now sets the classroom time at a minimum of 160 hours.

The Yoga Alliance's core curriculum for a 200-hour program (Registered Yoga School 200) covers techniques, training, and practice; anatomy and physiology; yoga humanities; and professional essentials. Each training submits their curriculum for review and approval or revision. There's some room for variety from program to program, but the intention is that the fundamentals be consistent across all Registered Yoga Schools (RYSs). Approval as an RYS is historically the last interaction between the school and the YA, apart from paying annual fees to maintain registry. Currently, there's no system of site visits or continued oversight of yoga schools that would parallel accreditation of colleges, or of technical programs like massage therapy schools. This may be a good thing, as government regulation can open an entirely new can of worms, choking the yoga field with bureaucracy and siphoning its profits while consolidating power in the hands of the few well-funded businesses that can afford to play by the new system.

That said, 200 hours is not that long, even with the recent upgrades to the teacher training requirements. In fact, 200 hours is just long enough to get the sense of the enormity of what you don't know. When you're doing an ecumenical overview of several styles, you'll sacrifice depth in service of breadth. By the end of our broad program at Carolina Yoga Company, for example, teachers have a sense of what they want to go on to study more deeply. In this way, a 200-hour teacher training is like the first two years of college. You'll be exposed to several different approaches to the practice. Some will resonate, some will not. Knowing what's out there and taking a good-faith survey of everything will guide you toward your major—toward the approach that makes the best sense for you, whether you develop and study it outside of formal education or move on to take an advanced studies teacher training.

At the end of your program, if you have met its requirements, you will graduate with a certificate from your school. If your teacher training was at a YA-affiliated school, you may be asked to evaluate how well the program met its stated goals—this is what the YA calls "social credentialing." You can then choose whether to register with the Yoga Alliance as a Registered Yoga Teacher at the 200-hour level (RYT 200).

There are various reasons why you might want to register or not care to. First, if you intend to teach at a gym, your hiring manager may want to see your RYT designation, or even your number and card, to show that you have been professionally trained. Second, you'll get guild rates on liability insurance, which we will discuss in chapter 5. Third, you'll get some nice perks: discounts at clothing stores and on services you might like to use for your class, like YogiTunes, which provides a license and platform for streaming music in class (something we'll discuss in chapter 7).

I have never been asked by a student for my Yoga Alliance registry number. And as a studio owner, I've never asked a teacher to prove affiliation with the Yoga Alliance. So should you register? It may not help you, but it isn't going to hurt you beyond putting a slight dent in your wallet (and this is a legitimate business expense, as we will discuss below), so it's worth trying. If you find it isn't at all useful, you simply won't renew.

300/500 Hours

Beyond the 200-hour level, YA-affiliated advanced studies programs can register as an RYS 300. After you complete the 300 or so hours of an advanced training from an RYS 300, you may add them to your previous 200-hour program and register as an RYT 500, denoting that you have had 500 hours of training.

If a 200-hour program is like the first two years of college, a 300-hour program is like the final years of college, when you're working to complete your major, possibly considering a minor, or taking fun classes in other areas that interest you. An advanced studies program can take you deep into a style that calls to you, which makes it a good complement to a broad 200-hour program. Or an RYS 300 can help you sharpen your skills to teach content of any kind—that's the way we structured our Carolina Yoga Company advanced studies program, which has modules on professionalism, classroom management, theming, language refinement, and much more.

How will you know when you are ready for an advanced studies program? When you're eager to learn more, not simply because it exists! It's useful to gain some teaching experience before undertaking your advanced training, especially if you're choosing a program like ours. That way every discussion of classroom issues will map onto your lived experience instead of being hypothetical and only intellectual. Many of these programs are modular, as ours is, so you can take the courses that interest you whether or not you eventually enroll in the full program.

1,000 Hours

If 500 hours isn't enough—and the deeper you go, the more 500 hours seems like a drop in the bucket—you can work toward a 1,000-hour training. These trainings are currently not affiliated with the Yoga Alliance, but they do provide some structure to your continuing education and might offer you a cohort of peers to grow with, one of the benefits of any teacher training. You'll find them at the Kripalu Center for Yoga and Health, Yoga Medicine, Dharma Yoga Center, and elsewhere. If you are ambitious and like to study in a system with formal benchmarks, a 1,000-hour training may give you the impetus to keep up your continuing study. Or you may be better served by focusing on ways to expand your yoga knowledge with complementary study. Ultimately, your students will be your best teachers, so don't let reaching for the next brass ring (1,000 hours! 1,500 hours!) keep you from doing the weekly work of showing up to teach the students who need you.

E-RYT Designation

The Yoga Alliance recognizes experienced teachers with the Experienced Registered Yoga Teacher designation (E-RYT). To qualify for the Experienced designation, a teacher needs at least 1,000 teaching hours after graduating from an RYS 200 and must have taught for two years or more since this graduation. For the E-RYT 500, the numbers double (but they include the first 1,000 hours and two years): You must have taught 2,000 hours, at least 500 of them after finishing your RYT 300/500 training, and be four years removed from your RYS 200 graduation.

Clear as mud? It's all outlined at yogaalliance.org. You may not care a bit about these designations, and your students likely won't either. But they may matter for your pay rate, and if you think you would like to lead a teacher training at a Yoga Alliance–registered school someday (Lead Trainers in Registered Yoga Schools must be E-RYT 500s), you should begin tracking your progress so you can apply once you're eligible.

Assess Your YTT Options

Take a look around your area, as well as places you could feasibly travel to, and make notes about your options for your first or your next YTT. Compare their formats to the format you think will best suit your available time and learning style. These prompts can help:

- How many hours do you have available per week to dedicate to training? If you don't have abundant free time, what will you need to let go of to make more time for training?

- Do you learn best by diving deep into material and working at it for several hours at a stretch? Or by letting yourself have time to digest what you've learned? Put another way: Do you like to binge-stream an entire season of a show, or would you rather space it out week by week?

- What financial resources do you have available for training?

- What logistical support do you have available, and what will you need to muster? This could be coverage at your day job, child or pet care, and the like.

For each program, list:

- Program name:

- Format (e.g., weekend, intensive) and dates:

- Program cost:

- Other costs, like travel or room and board:

Writing this out will probably show you that you are drawn toward a particular program. If you really feel you can't make up your mind between two comparable options, flip a coin. Your reaction to the coin toss—not the result itself—might show you where your heart lies.

QUESTIONS TO ASK ABOUT YOUR PROSPECTIVE TEACHER TRAINING

If you feel the calling, it's better to choose a teacher training that meets most of your requirements rather than waiting for the "perfect" option. This is just the start of your education as a teacher, and waiting for the ideal conditions, schedule, or location may mean you never undertake the journey at all. Don't let perfect be the enemy of good enough. That said, you'll want satisfying answers to these questions.

Can I take a class from the lead teacher(s)?

This is an important first step in your research. You need not want to teach like the lead teacher or teachers at the school, but being able to understand their communication styles is critical. Better still than taking a class is taking a workshop where the lead teacher explains not just what to do but also how and why, since how and why is a lot of the material that is taught in YTT. Do your research. If you can't take a class in person with the lead teachers, ask if there's video of them online. It'd be smart to have a quick chat before or after this class, or to set up a phone call so you can ask all your questions about the program.

What do students find the most challenging part of training?

Listen carefully to the answer to this question and compare it to what you personally expect to find difficult in the training. Consider how you would handle this challenge. Are you nervous speaking in front of a crowd? Your first practice teach might be tough. Do you anticipate trouble in a long day of asana practice? Ask the school representative how students have handled fatigue in the past.

How long has this program and this particular format been offered?

New is not necessarily bad—trainers have extra enthusiasm for the first round or two of their training. Some trainings have been running for years like a well-oiled machine; others have recently been overhauled or have had a change of teacher. Be sure you feel that the format you're considering is going to work for you.

What does any given day in YTT look like?

Getting a sense of the schedule will help you determine whether it is the right environment for your learning style. It's also useful to know what proportion of the day is spent on asana, lecture, chanting, and other activities. If some or all of the program is online, how much engagement and attention do students get? You will not grow as a teacher unless you get specific feedback.

How do you handle physical limitations?

Some programs want incoming students to be able to press to wheel pose and do a handstand away from the wall. If this turns you off, that's not the program for you! Many other programs are happy to work with physical limitations. I always tell our prospective students that they will be more sympathetic and empathetic teachers by needing to work around their own personal issues in asana. We've had students from fifteen to seventy-something in our training, and in each group there's someone with a reason to sit and watch a given asana practice instead of participating. It's not a problem. Sometimes watching is a better teacher than doing.

What is a typical next step for your graduates?

They may audition for the studio that hosts the training or for other studios, be encouraged to join the work-study program, or be upsold to a new training. Listen for an honest answer and ask yourself whether it meshes with your vision for your career.

Can I talk to some recent graduates? Can I see them teach?

We ask prospective teacher trainees to come to a class with me, where there is usually at least one current YTT student as well as alumni. I love connecting them, so the prospective student can get a recent graduate's take on the program.

Our trainees also lead a $5 community class to gain practice teaching, and we encourage those who are considering our program to attend one or more of these, so that they can get a sense both of what our students do well and also of where their own teaching skills might be during or just after YTT.

Look through the studio's teacher biographies to find those who graduated from the program, and plan to attend their classes and ask questions about their path and their experience in the program.

What if I have to miss time?

You'll have to make it up, and different programs approach this differently. In a weekend program, there is often someone who can't bow out of, say, a family wedding; in a weekday program, parents may find themselves suddenly stuck at home with a sick child. Many programs charge an hourly rate for makeups, because to meet the Yoga Alliance standards—if your targeted training does—you must hit the minimum number of contact hours.

What is your refund policy?

This should be clearly stated on the training's website; if not, be sure to ask. Teacher training costs a lot for the student and is an important part of a studio's revenue, so they may not offer refunds but instead give you credit toward a future training. And there are some circumstances where a student is asked to leave a training, so it might be good to ask if this has been an issue and on what grounds students are expelled. (This should be a reassuring discussion, not a terrifying one.)

> **Take Scouting Visit Notes**

Make notes on the answers you get to these questions from your prospective schools.

- ▶ Can I take a class from the lead teacher(s)?
- ▶ What do students find the most challenging part of training?
- ▶ How long has this program and this particular format been offered?
- ▶ What does any given day in YTT look like?
- ▶ How do you handle physical limitations?
- ▶ What is a typical next step for your graduates?
- ▶ Can I talk to some recent graduates? Can I see them teach?
- ▶ What if I have to miss time?
- ▶ What is your refund policy?

CONTINUING STUDENTHOOD

Classes

Your very best training will come from your students. You'll see whether and how your cues land with them. They'll surprise you with special needs that you'll have to scramble to meet, which will make you better prepared the next time something similar happens. The stranger the places you teach, the fewer the props, and the more constraints your students have, the more you will learn. Go out and teach!

At the same time, you *must* continue to take classes. Look for a balance of consistency and variety here. Choose one or two teachers with whom you'll study regularly—at least once a month, and maybe once a week—so that you may further your understanding of that teacher's approach. This gives you depth. But also choose a wide range of teachers you'll study with occasionally, so that your understanding of yoga is not just deep but also broad. Every teacher has something to offer you. Sometimes it's a turn of phrase, or a new approach to a familiar shape. Sometimes it's a lesson in what not to do. The teachers that most push your buttons may have the most to teach you about what you value in a class and in an instructor.

Every trip to a new place is a new opportunity to start afresh as a student. Find a local studio and observe how easy or difficult it is to navigate their website to choose a class. Watch the process as you park, walk in, pay for the class, and get centered. How does the teacher welcome you? How do their cues land? How is the transition out of class? In every experience, you'll find a rose and some thorns, and taking careful note of the negatives will help you find ways to enhance your students' experience. Keep a journal or a notes file and write down what you learn in each class you go to.

If you always only practice on your own, you are like a terminal pond: There is no incoming source of fresh water to refill you. Remaining a student keeps you from being a closed system. Regular infusion of fresh teaching, poses, transitions, language, and music will keep you developing as a teacher.

Workshops

In addition to your own regular class attendance and ongoing self-study, it's good to take workshops that expand your understanding of yoga and mindfulness. If you already do this, it's good to reflect on what you've been learning. If you've been drawn exclusively to workshops that confirm what you already believe, try to find some that will challenge you. What are the weaker spots in your knowledge, and how can you shore them up with continuing study?

If you have been trained in a power or flow style of yoga, you might seek training in alignment-based styles; or in yin, restorative, or gentle yoga; or in therapeutics; or in the subtle body. If you've been flummoxed by how to handle older students with limited mobility, seek a training on yoga for healthy aging or yoga for seniors. If you feel like your sequencing has hit a rut, look for trainings to freshen it. And at any point, deepening your understanding of anatomy and kinesiology will make you a better teacher.

Depending on where you live, you may have a host of workshops to choose from locally or regionally. Or maybe you'll make a point to travel occasionally to a yoga center like Kripalu in western Massachusetts, or the 1440 Multiversity in Santa Cruz, California. Increasingly, you can take wonderful trainings online in a multitude of disciplines. Ask your colleagues and your mentors what has been useful to them.

Challenge yourself with your choices. If a workshop is simply affirming your beliefs, it's wasting your time and isn't teaching you anything. There has to be a stretch for you to integrate new information. This might lead you to a new specialization.

Specialties

Yoga is for everyone, and specialty training in how to work with various populations will both help you serve students and make you stand out as a professional.

The Yoga Alliance recognizes two specialties with acronyms of their own: prenatal yoga and children's yoga. To become a Registered Prenatal Yoga Teacher (RPYT), you'd complete a 200-hour training and an 85-hour prenatal training that is registered with the Yoga Alliance (look for the acronym RPYS, Registered Prenatal Yoga School), then document 30 hours of experience after the specialty training. Similarly, for children's yoga, the acronyms are RCYT and RCYS, and the RCYS program must last 95 hours on top of your 200-hour training. But you need not follow this system to be a good prenatal yoga or kids' yoga teacher—you are likely to find several alternative trainings that equip you with the basics.

At the other end of the life span spectrum is yoga for seniors. Carol Krucoff and Kimberly Carson's program at Duke Integrative Medicine is an especially well-researched one based on updated scientific evidence; see yoga4seniors.com. You could also explore chair yoga, yoga for cancer patients and survivors, yoga for various conditions like arthritis or multiple sclerosis—your students and your interests can guide you toward the trainings that will suit you best.

Beyond these age-specific specialties sanctioned by the Yoga Alliance, there is a wide world of wonderful resources to explore after your initial yoga teacher training. Many will help you specialize in a particular group of students or a particular style of yoga, as we've seen. Some will offer you a particular way to help whoever is in your class. Here are some approaches that offer you a lens you can apply to any open class.

▶ Bigger bodies: Anna Guest-Jelley's Curvy Yoga program, curvyyoga.com
▶ Social justice: Michelle Cassandra Johnson's Skill in Action and Dismantling Racism trainings; see michellecjohnson.com
▶ Trauma: David Emerson's work, traumasensitiveyoga.com

You can also seek out programs for teaching yoga to veterans or to the differently abled—any population that you feel you can help. Here's where you can truly live your yoga, bringing its benefits beyond the studio walls and into your community.

Certifications

Teachers can also confer certifications of their own design, as I do with my Sage Yoga for Athletes program. Who granted me the power to certify others? Well: I did! I set the standards, I work directly with students to be sure they display mastery of the material, and I certify them. What does that mean? Simply that they have my seal of approval. This can matter for gyms or teams, and it offers my international students a chance to say they are the only certified Sage Yoga for Athletes teacher in their home country, if the country is small enough. I choose my workshop assistants from these certified teachers, and I always connect them with opportunities when I can, such as pointing journalists seeking a quote their way.

If you are drawn to a training that offers a certificate, don't be shy to ask about the authority behind that certificate and what doors the certificate might open for you. And always ask for references—any good trainer will be happy to connect you to other students who have gone through the program.

The International Association of Yoga Therapists

The International Association of Yoga Therapists, or IAYT, is an organization of yoga therapists, specialized teachers who typically work one-on-one with clients toward health-based outcomes and improvements. As such, the work combines elements of yoga teaching, counseling, and physical therapy. The IAYT is separate from the Yoga Alliance, which now disallows use of the terms "yoga therapy" and "yoga therapist" for RYTs describing their work. Read about the IAYT's certification process and about the field of yoga therapy at iayt.org.

Repeating Trainings

Just like people go back to school and change careers, people can and do take multiple teacher trainings. My two closest collaborators have done just that. Alexandra DeSiato, who has cowritten two books with me, took a wonderful Prana Vinyasa Flow teacher training, in which she dove deep into this particular style, originated by Shiva Rea. Then she went through the Carolina Yoga Company 200-hour program, which offers a broader perspective. The combination of the two gave her both a wide and a deep view of the practice and how to teach.

Jenni Tarma, who co-teaches yoga teacher trainings with me, has completed two advanced teacher trainings. One is the Yoga Medicine program developed by Tiffany Cruikshank, which has a very strong focus on anatomy. The other is the advanced studies program led by Jules Mitchell, a biomechanist. These complementary programs have made Jenni an expert on anatomy, and she has enhanced this awareness by adding coaching certifications from the Road Runners Club of America and CrossFit.

Learning is a lifelong process. If you're reading this book as an experienced teacher feeling stale, or looking to reach the next level in your career, consider jumping off your current track and onto another one. Would a fresh training give you a new viewpoint? If you were taught in an alignment-based school, would you benefit from studying flow yoga, and vice versa? (I think so!) Or would picking up study in a specialty, like yin or restorative or yoga for seniors, juice you up anew for your teaching?

My Experience

Shortly after finishing my 200-hour training, I moved through the Spinning indoor cycling certification process, eventually reaching Star 3, their top tier of education. This got me thinking about how yoga and cycling went together. It also got me a gig teaching indoor cycling at a very nice wellness center, where I also taught yoga. Once a week, I did the two together: an hour of cycling, followed by 45 minutes of yoga. Spinning's take on indoor cycling is to make it as road-specific as possible: There's less all-out sprinting and more nuance. As a road rider and triathlete, I bought in. But the gym students were used to a more all-out style, and it took quite some time—easily a year—for me to find my tribe. This was a great lesson: Do what you believe in, explain clearly why you believe it, and your people will find you.

I then moved into trainings in endurance sport coaching: USA Triathlon, USA Cycling, and the Road Runners Club of America. Each of these programs taught me more about exercise physiology and psychology, and each informed not only my own training but also my yoga teaching. I spent several years coaching runners, road and mountain bike riders, and triathletes, with some of my clients reaching the world championship levels in their sports and others finishing 100-mile races. This was rewarding work but also a big energetic output, similar to teaching private yoga lessons. I felt 100 percent responsible for each client's success. Now that I'm busy at the studio, I've phased out this work, though I still advise my former clients as they coach themselves.

These experiences were key research. They taught me a lot about how the body and mind work, and this directly helped me as a yoga teacher. They also gave me authority to develop my niche in teaching yoga to athletes. What are your passions, and how can you follow them?

OTHER MOVEMENT STYLES

To keep your movement practice fresh and avoid yoga burnout, make a point of trying other modalities, like Pilates, Gyrotonics, Feldenkrais, and so on. Or study martial arts: Karate, Krav Maga, Judo. These modalities will take a different path up the mountain of body awareness and mindful movement, and studying them will inform your yoga practice and keep your teaching fresh.

To learn more about the body, and to deepen your expertise in hands-on assists, take an introductory course in massage—or a full massage training. In addition to owning Carolina Yoga Company, my business partner and I own a massage school, Carolina Massage Institute. Several of our graduates have completed yoga teacher training and actively teach, and some of our yoga teacher trainees have completed the massage program.

Thai Yoga Massage, sometimes called Thai Partner Yoga or Thai Assisted Stretching, is another good arrow to have in your quiver. You'll be an expert at savasana assists with that certification under your belt. Depending on state licensure rules, you may or may not be able to use the word "massage" when promoting this work, but regardless of the rules around the nomenclature, it's a great technique to bring into your yoga classroom and private lessons.

Further, take a cadaver dissection course or anatomy class at your local community college. There are several offerings of cadaver dissection for body workers and movement teachers. I did a six-day lab with Gil Hedley; several of my colleagues have completed a lab with Tiffany Cruikshank's Yoga Medicine program. These programs are awesome in the original sense of the word: They will put you in awe of the human form, the gift of the donors, and the profound learning that occurs with a deep exploration of the body. While there are nice virtual-reality programs for the squeamish, there is nothing like being able to dissect a cadaver using your own hands and eyes.

The Functional Movement Screen (FMS) is a battery of tests that personal trainers, athletic trainers, and strength and conditioning coaches use to identify imbalances in their athletes. Taking a one-day training or the online course (functionalmovement.com) in how to administer the tests will give you a language for talking to trainers and coaches. Better yet, it will give you an assessment to use at the start of private lessons, so that you can begin by shoring up your clients' weak spots. I highly recommend that you look into this training or similar ones. While you might not wind up using the tests in the screen as is, they will get you thinking about how to assess your students' bodies so that they can find better balance through yoga.

In a different vein, try classes in stand-up comedy, improvisational theater, storytelling, cooking, sewing, brewing, conversational Mandarin—anything that puts you into a student's mind and presents you with a learning curve. All of these will make you a more present, sympathetic, and empathetic teacher. And all of them will guide you toward better self-awareness, the goal of yoga. Let's explore your self-awareness and begin to articulate a vision for your career, whatever stage it's in.

3

Clarify Your Vision

· ·

IF YOU FIND THIS BOOK before you embark on a teacher training, wonderful! You can enter your YTT clear-eyed about the role that yoga and the teaching of it can fill in your life, and after YTT you can start to craft the career you want. But at any and every point in your teaching journey, it's helpful to assess where you are, where you want to be, and how best to help yourself and your students. In this chapter, you'll be prompted to think through what brought you to yoga and what you can bring to it, to articulate the cardinal rules you believe about yoga and teaching, to question and crystallize those rules, and to set or revise a vision for your work as a professional yoga teacher.

RECOGNIZE YOUR BACKSTORY: FIND YOUR WHY

As I mentioned in the preface, I come from a family of educators, and I came to yoga right after seven years of graduate school, during five of which I was teaching English writing and literature. This backstory informed my desire to teach yoga, because I could see myself pretty easily in the seat of the teacher. It also informed my vision of the kind of teacher I wanted to be, in part because I knew the kind of teacher I was in the college English classroom: a guide who had rather recently learned to analyze the same texts the class was reading, and whose fresh experience was re-formed in the process of teaching. Similarly, I began as a yoga teacher working with people like me: endurance athletes who felt tight and tired and wondered whether yoga might both ease their pains and develop their mental strength. Having recently recognized the ways yoga helped my own training, I was equipped to help students who had a similar backstory. I could have had a parallel career as a prenatal yoga teacher, or a yoga-for-parents teacher, as the experience of pregnancy, childbirth, and parenting was also very fresh for me as I began teaching.

Lately, I've been working in yoga for healthy aging (more on this in my *Lifelong Yoga*, cowritten with Alexandra DeSiato) and doable core moves based on my own love of taking creative Pilates classes that put a contemporary spin on the classical moves—this became my Core Strength for Real People video series. Again, my own interests and experiences have informed my teaching. And so should yours! As we know, you need to be you, not Bryan and not Sage. Your authentic backstory will give you a sense of your why and point you to what kind of teacher you want to be.

Write Your Backstory

Consider and list the experiences you have had that brought you to yoga—was it a pregnancy, a desire to get in shape, a need for downtime and centering, or something else? Write a little about these experiences.

Now think of experiences you've had in the seat of the teacher. These need not be in a classroom setting; perhaps you've been a scout leader, a team captain, or a babysitter. What attitude did you adopt in these situations? What kind of teacher do you have experience being?

Finally, write about what kind of teacher this backstory has set you up to be.

FIND YOUR WHO AND YOUR WHAT

Now that you've reflected on the path that's brought you to this point, think about who your students are. This is a useful exercise whether or not you are already teaching.

Find Your Audience

While you'll often be adapting to teach the students who are in the room, especially if you're teaching open classes in person, you'll find the greatest ease and success by spending some time envisioning your ideal audience. This way, you can take next steps toward working with the people who will most benefit from what you have to teach and how you teach it.

Write a little in response to these prompts: Who are your students? Whom do you naturally relate to? Middle school teachers, for example, are a special crew. With whom do you share your happiest social events? Is it gardeners, athletes, chess players, children, your elders?

Only once you are clear on your audience can you see what best to teach them. To paraphrase the master teacher Cyndi Lee, your role is not to teach your students what you know—it's to teach them what they *don't* know.

Find Your Content

To determine what your students need to know, first determine your audience. Then ask yourself, "What is a problem this audience has?" To drill down more: Where does this audience exist, what activities do they do—or how and why are they inactive—and what patterns do people in this audience develop in mind and body? How can these patterns become a problem? How can yoga solve that problem?

For example, let's say your audience is long-haul truckers. They spend many hours each day sitting with their arms reaching forward, and with their left arms on the windowsill and their right hands on the wheel. They use their right legs and their left legs in different ways to operate the clutch and gas pedals. Think of the imbalances this work accrues, and how most truckers don't have the time for or access to gyms or trails to get in a post-drive workout or hike.

In this example, you might design a beginner-friendly but active practice that gets the truckers moving and draws their attention to how the right and left sides of their bodies might feel different, and how the front of their bodies may seem tighter than the back. This practice would include some passive backbends to stretch the front, and some active backbends to strengthen the back.

Aha! Suddenly this example doesn't seem so esoteric. You may not find yourself teaching a room full of long-haul truckers, but you will likely have a room full of students who spend much of their day sitting at a desk, and sitting in a car or train on the way to and from work. Their needs will be similar.

Beyond the physical, what are the mental demands on your audience? Do they need to spend a lot of time focused on one thing—what in yoga we would call *dharana* (intense concentration)? Or do they need to spend a lot of time in presence, aware of many things at once? We'd call that *diyana* (meditative awareness). Depending on these demands, you might include various breath exercises, teach mantra, explain and challenge *drishti* (focused gaze), or make other choices to give your students what they need.

If you're teaching an open class, you may not have a very clear grasp of who your audience is week to week. But if you watch your students closely, you'll be able to see trends. If you teach at a gym, for example, you may have a wide range of students. But depending on your class time and title, you may find that your students tend to be weightlifters, or cardiac rehab patients, or moms taking advantage of the free childcare to take some time for themselves. Once you identify these trends, you'll be able to ask yourself what problem this audience has, and how you can offer yoga to solve it.

Find Your Message

The lessons yoga has taught you are the very ones you'll be teaching your students. Write a little about your three or four biggest takeaways from yoga. I imagine you'll find they are big life lessons—not "it helps to flex your foot in *x* pose" but "you're capable of more than you think" or "we all hold way more tension than we are aware of, and stillness is often the best way to realize this and to dissolve it."

Now, could you distill these lessons to a short phrase like, "Find the balance between effort and ease," or "Find the right breath for now," or "Do less," or "Hang on"? These will be your guiding principles and messages as a teacher. Come back to them often.

WHAT ARE THE RULES?

New yoga teachers like rules. This makes sense: If you were in your first semester of cooking school, you'd want to know the rules, too! But once you're versed in what has been presented to you as the rules of alignment and sequencing (and you're about to see that I believe there are very few hard-and-fast rules), you'll need to begin an educated questioning of these rules. In what cases do they admit exception? Why are the rules imposed in the first case? Who came up with them, who enforces them, and what would happen if they were broken?

This goes not only for alignment and sequencing but also for every element of your class. To guide you about when to follow and when consciously to break the rules, consider the context. The cooking analogy holds up here.

Are you teaching at a studio with a specific style, and if so, what is expected of you? This would be clearly communicated in a manual and in your training. In the cooking analogy, this is like working at a franchise. Part of the appeal of McDonald's or Starbucks, for example, is that you can walk into one anywhere and expect to order the same familiar items and to receive them prepared in the same familiar way.

But if you are cooking at your own place, and especially if you are given free rein either explicitly (you have created and are hosting a class of your own) or implicitly (you are an independent contractor—we'll cover this later on), you'll have much more room to improvise your recipes and cook based on what is in season and what your students' palates crave. You'll still need to follow the few rules that universally help with student safety, just as you'd need to follow food safety laws regardless of where you're cooking. But you'll have a lot more freedom of expression.

Yoga spent centuries as an oral culture, passed from teacher to student. Many of the rules have been repeated this way for generations. As a student and a new teacher, you will find yourself repeating them. This is only natural: You respect your teachers, you trust that what they say is because they have your best interests at heart, and you know you have your own students' best interests at heart, too. But once you have gained some comfort with the basic elements of class, undertake a reasoned investigation of what rules you're conferring on your students, and whether they apply. Don't simply repeat things because they're what you've heard. Instead, offer them because they have been proven through your own study and practice. Your experience and your curiosity should guide you.

For example, you've likely heard that in tree pose, students should never rest their raised-leg foot against their standing-leg knee. Why not? Try it now. Did you feel your chakras spin in the wrong direction? Of course not. If your knee isn't capable of handling the light stress of a foot resting against it, you'll be in trouble when you step off a curb and torque it, or when an enthusiastic dog or child runs into you.

Similarly, you may have been taught your feet should be in a particular arrangement for Warrior I, and another very particular arrangement for Warrior II and similar poses. (To further confound things, different styles can dictate different but exact placement of your feet.) Why? Have you challenged your teacher for a response? Have you considered how unique morphology—each individual's different skeleton, especially the intersection of the pelvis and the femur at the hip joint—might demand a different alignment? Start asking questions like this of yourself, your teachers, and, when appropriate, your students. How does it feel to try things a different way?

Safety in Class Is Like Food Safety

New teachers are often invested in "the rules," wanting to make sure they get everything right. Similarly, new parents are terrified about caring for their fragile infants, but they quickly learn that babies are durable. So are your students. As long as they aren't wildly flailing to kick into a headstand, they are likely safe, and a slight deviation from the Platonic ideal of a pose may actually be safer for a student, given their unique body. No one wants to feel like a failure in a yoga class; an overemphasis on the "right" way to do a pose can set up students, especially new students, to feel like they aren't good at yoga.

Once again, a food analogy comes to bear. Imagine you are preparing a buffet. There are some important food safety rules to follow to prevent poisoning your guests: Wash vegetables well; cook poultry and pork to indicated temperatures; keep hot foods hot and cold foods cold; don't leave anything out at room temperature for very long. Within the context of these rules, you're setting out what you think will be palatable to your guests. And they can choose what to put on their plates.

Perhaps one of these guests has a food allergy. It would be important for them to avoid eating the foods that they are allergic to, and it would be up to you as the cook to answer any questions they have about the ingredients and preparation so they can make an informed decision. If the party is small and you have advance notice, you can prepare an alternative, just as you would if you were teaching a private lesson and knew your student had some injuries to work around. But in the context of a large gathering, there will be enough other offerings on the table that a guest with an allergy can skip the items that would sicken them and still leave satisfied.

My Actual Rules

In my experience over many years of teaching, virtually everything I once believed to be a clear-cut truth about yoga has proved to be more nuanced. Through years of study of yoga, anatomy, and exercise physiology while working to keep an open mind, here are my currently held beliefs.

1. Be clear on why you're doing what you're doing. Constantly ask *why*. To have an efficient and specific practice, you should be able to justify any movement, exercise, or technique you are doing. "For fun!" is a fine reason.
2. No movement is inherently bad or wrong. Doing *any* movement too much will lead to injury. Find the appropriate dose of any stress you choose. Too little and there won't be change; too much and you will break down.
3. Students are responsible for caring for their needs. Everything I mention as a teacher is a suggestion; students must make their own choices about whether to take any shape or movement, and students must choose the right amount for their own bodies.

And that's it. Three rules!

Articulate Your Rules

What do you consider the actual rules or cardinal rules of yoga, and in particular, of asana practice? List them.

Now to each item on the list, add a reason why you believe these. It's OK to write, "I think your raised-arm palm should face forward in triangle pose. Why? Because my teacher said so." Only by questioning the origin of your long-held beliefs can you make informed choices about whether they are true now.

Finally, do some research on whether they hold up. Are there peer-reviewed studies that support your beliefs? Do different styles take alternative approaches that contradict your rules? What would it be like to try these approaches? Be open.

IMPOSTER SYNDROME

A creeping sense that you are a phony goes hand in hand with the destabilization that comes from questioning your beliefs. Our yoga teacher trainees often ask me, "When did you stop feeling like a fraud?" The question makes me smile, because it presumes that I've ever stopped. Some days, I still feel like I'm not experienced enough, or perky enough, or whatever enough to lead my students. And I do it anyway. If I taught only when I was in the perfect mood to teach, I wouldn't teach at all.

Imposter syndrome is real, particularly for women. My best advice is to fake it until you make it. With luck, you'll feel more authoritative over time. But recognize that some days you won't. On those days, do it anyway. It can help to imagine you are playing a role—because, in a way, you are. Don't expect to feel perfectly authentic; do focus on what your students need: a teacher to guide them in breath and movement.

You don't need to know it all, you just need to have a plan and guide your students. Teaching yoga isn't brain surgery or landing a jet plane. Keep it simple, smile, and leave lots of time for students to go inward. Don't fill every moment with the sound of your voice out of a desire to prove your worth! Instead, issue a clear direction, then be quiet and let the students enjoy their practice.

On the other hand: Often students *say* they want a 6:00 AM class, but they really mean they want to be the kind of person who shows up to a 6:00 AM class. (More than once, we've added early classes to the studio schedule because of student demand, and then . . . crickets.) The same thing can apply to yoga teacher trainees. They want to be the kind of person who would wholeheartedly embrace yoga and float through teacher training. They want to be the kind of person who will confidently fill the seat of the teacher. Taking a good look at your motivation and setting realistic expectations will ensure that you get the most out of your teacher training experience and, as your career progresses, your experience as a professional yoga teacher. You will feel more authentic to your vision when you are able to articulate your vision with clear intentions and goals.

With the recognition that teaching yoga is, for most of us, a way to give back and a side gig that complements our primary work, you will want to make wise plans about how your career can grow as a complement to your other commitments. Keep your eyes wide open about the time you have to devote to teaching and the income you will need to receive. This will guide you to smart choices about what jobs you take. This workbook exercise will help.

Clarify Your Intentions and Goals

Being very clear on both intentions and goals will help you make choices in any situation, from running a marathon to designing your career. I consider intentions to be about the inner process—the feelings you want to have as you undertake and complete a project, from running a marathon to finishing yoga teacher training to leading a single class. Intentions are about the process. Goals, on the other hand, are about the outcome. These might include hitting a particular time in the marathon, or earning a certain amount per class as a yoga teacher.

Take some time to journal about and list your *intentions* for becoming a yoga teacher. Ask yourself:

▶ What feelings come up for me around the role of yoga teacher?

▶ What qualities does a good yoga teacher demonstrate?

▶ How do I want to show up for my students?

▶ How do I want my students to feel after class with me?

Given what you've written, write yourself a mission statement, an overarching declaration of your intention as a teacher of yoga. Here's mine:

I use the privilege of my education and varied experiences by sharing freely from what I have learned to benefit my students.

Now consider your *goals*, remembering that these are external, public, and measurable. These might build on the goals you noted in chapter 1, or you might have already thought about going in new directions. Ask yourself:

▶ Given my other work, health, and family obligations, how many hours a week can I spend practicing yoga?

▶ Given my other work, health, and family obligations, how many hours a week can I reasonably spend *teaching* yoga?

▶ How many of those hours would be spent leading a live class? How many hours would be spent online and creating content?

▶ What would it take, either in money or in benefits (like free gym membership or free studio classes), for me to feel like my time is fully valued?

▶ Recognizing that I have to start somewhere, how long am I willing to work toward this fair-value goal?

▶ And, most critically:

▶ What is the first next step toward this goal?

Your answer to this next-step question will begin to structure your action plan. Perhaps it's researching teacher trainings, or a new studio you want to apply to teach for, or asking for a raise. Write out this step, and the next, and the next, until you hit a natural endpoint. (For more on project management along these lines, read David Allen's *Getting Things Done*.)

As you did in chapter 1, set yourself reminders to check in on these goals. Review them at least quarterly or—better yet—once a month. When you do these regular checkups, you might find that a goal isn't relevant anymore, so revise as necessary. Sometimes a big goal needs to be broken down into smaller parts. And sometimes a goal needs to be postponed while you focus on the smaller next steps that will eventually take you there.

One of your goals likely includes furthering your career as a yoga teacher. I imagine you're planning to start teaching or developing a presence online, or you want to up your game, or you feel like you're stagnating and want a fresh infusion of energy for your teaching. Let's take a look at how you can define and promote yourself so students find you and can benefit from what you have to offer.

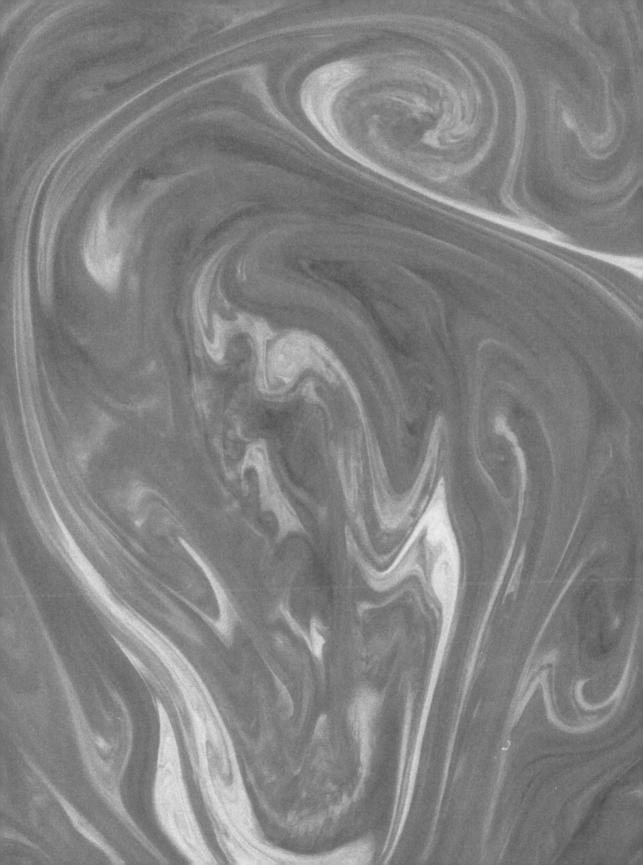

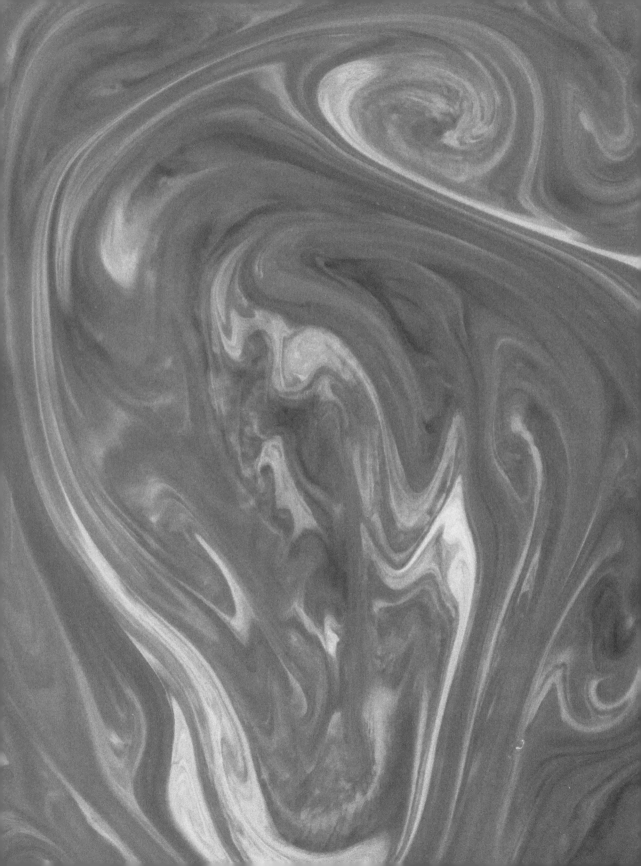

PART 2

Building Your Career

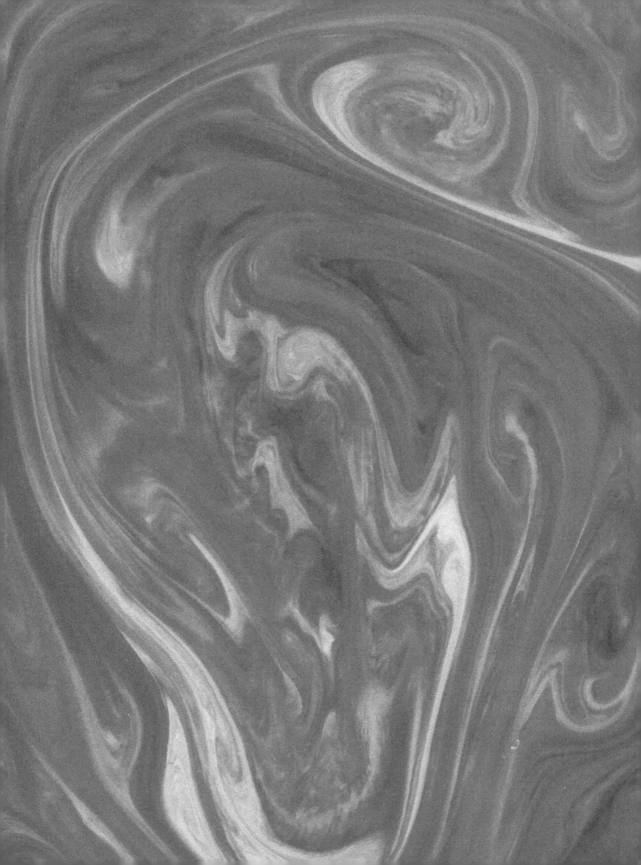

4

Promotion

. . . .

SINCE PROMOTION WILL BE an ongoing feature of your career as a yoga teacher, it's worth thinking about it early on and revisiting it often. When you're first getting started, figuring out your marketing and promotion strategy will help you clarify who you are and establish a presence that can land you your first jobs. It's a natural next step after articulating your motivation and your visions. And it's an important thing to revisit when you're feeling too busy, not busy enough, or stale in your practice and teaching. Some of what you'll find in this chapter will be appropriate and necessary for you right now; other actions that I'll suggest will come down the road once you've landed your first or next teaching job. Be sure to revisit these steps regularly—the timeline in the appendix will help keep you on track. Putting a little bit of time in monthly will keep your promotion up-to-date and yield you the best results.

For your promotion, you'll need various *assets*. These are the materials that specify exactly who you are. They include written content, photos and videos, and other images: from a logo, if you choose to have one, to a color palette, to fonts. Since you know who you are—or since you're getting to the heart of it through your yoga practice—it makes sense to start by writing your teaching biography.

DEVELOP A BIOGRAPHY

Whether you are building your website or teaching at a gym, studio, or festival, you will need a good biography. Start with role models. Look online at the bios of your favorite teachers, both those with a national visibility, with whom you may have studied online or at a workshop or festival, and the local luminaries. What qualities do good bios have in common? A good biography is as much about the reader as it is about the teacher, making it clear how people will feel after taking a class or a workshop from the teacher. It should show personality rather than simply listing credentials. It doesn't need to be cutesy, but it does need to convey the essence of the teacher.

Here's my short bio that appears on the teacher page of my studio site.

As an athlete, endurance sports coach, and continuing student of yoga, Sage Rountree understands the trickiness of balancing training and a yoga practice. Sage's classes emphasize intention and efficiency—using the right form and the right breath for the task at hand. There's plenty of attention to core, the hips, and using the body, breath, and mind to focus. An Experienced Registered Yoga Teacher with the Yoga Alliance at the highest level (E-RYT 500), Sage has over sixteen years' experience teaching yoga to students of all levels and backgrounds, including several UNC teams and Coach Roy Williams. Co-owner of the studio, director of our teacher trainings, and the author of nine books, including The Athlete's Guide to Yoga, Everyday Yoga, Lifelong Yoga, Teaching Yoga Beyond the Poses, *and* The Professional Yoga Teacher's Handbook, *Sage has also written for* Yoga Journal, Runner's World, Lava Magazine, *and* USA Triathlon Magazine.

While it ends with a curriculum vitae–style rundown of my published works, it gives an overview of what students can expect from my classes, then grounds my work in the context of our university town, where the basketball coach is a celebrity. To see other examples of a range of biography lengths and focuses, you'll find my media kit at yogateacherhandbook.com.

Draft Your Bio

Answer these questions, going into as much detail as you like. Then cull the best sentences and phrases from your answers and distill them into a one- or two-paragraph biography.

- ▶ What first brought you to yoga? What were your revelations from your first few classes?

- ▶ What does yoga mean to you?

- ▶ Who and what have been your greatest teachers? While you may be tempted to simply list everyone you've ever studied with, can you think outside the box?

- ▶ How has your practice changed over the years?

- ▶ How do you want students to feel in your class? How do you want them to feel after your class? What would you like to hear them say to each other on the way out the door?

RÉSUMÉ

If you don't already have one, get to work on a yoga résumé; if you have one, update it now. This is different from your day-job work résumé, as it's not a comprehensive catalog of all of your work experience but a précis of only what's relevant to yoga. Your background in dance or gymnastics or improv theater would go on here; your work as a hotel reception desk agent or a waiter could arguably appear on your yoga résumé, as it's customer service; the work-study you did in the music library in college or your time scooping ice cream as a teenager isn't relevant.

Create a document now, save it in the cloud, and add to it as you grow as a teacher. You might even find yourself subtracting items that you used to round out the résumé at the start of your career, but which have now been superseded. At the top, give your name and contact information, including your web page and, if relevant, your yoga-related social media handles. Then add these sections.

Education and Training

If you completed college or graduate school with a major in a yoga-related or caregiving field (nursing, dance, exercise physiology, religion, philosophy, psychology), list it. You do not need to list non–yoga-related education, like your major in statistics or your high school.

If you have taken a 200-hour or a 300-hour teacher training, a children's yoga or a prenatal yoga training, list it by name with the dates completed. When relevant, give the lead teachers' names. If there is a particular slant to your training—it's in a branded style of yoga, or focused on yin or therapeutics or kirtan or something specific—add it.

If you have taken continuing education workshops, or a workshop with a notable teacher, add it here, with the teacher's name, workshop title, location and date, and a word about content, if it would be helpful.

Teaching Experience

If you're already teaching yoga, list your classes here, with start and—when relevant— end dates. If you taught at a unique time, like 5:30 AM or Sundays at 8:00 PM, or a prime-time spot like Tuesdays at 6:00 PM or Saturdays at 10:00 AM, add that, as it will let your hiring manager know you're flexible and capable.

If you've been teaching for a long time, you need not list every class, just the highlights. List the locations where you've taught, with a line or two about the classes you led.

If you haven't started teaching yet, you may need to reach to fill your teaching experience section. That's OK! You probably have taught as part of your teacher training: Describe that. Did you lead ten-minute classes? Sixty-minute classes? Community classes? Did you volunteer to practice on groups of friends and family? Show that you are actively creating opportunities for teaching.

Relevant Skills

If you've been involved with running a studio in any capacity, from sweeping floors to stocking bathrooms to checking in students to selling retail, list it here. If you have familiarity with studio management or scheduling software like MindBody Online, Wellness Living, Tula, or Vagaro, highlight that with a line or two about what kind of work you did in the software (class check-in, appointments, contracts).

If you have video production experience, detail it. If you have skill in a foreign language, particularly if you can teach yoga in Spanish or another common language, add it here. Likewise, add CPR/AED certifications, first aid skills, or other special skills.

References

Enlist three references. These can include the studio manager or owner where you're teaching, if you are; your teacher trainer or other yoga mentor; and a well-spoken student who's taken your class regularly. If you are not teaching yet, list a colleague from teacher training who can speak about your development and growth as a teacher. Check with each of these individuals to confirm they are willing to give you a positive recommendation before listing them as references.

Bio and Headshot

Include a one-paragraph bio that the studio can use (as you've drafted in the previous workbook exercise), and consider adding a headshot. While this would be against employment law for an office job at a major corporation, it's common in the arts. If you're applying to teach at a particular studio, model your bio and headshot on those you'll find at their website. The idea is to make it as easy as possible for your hiring manager to see you fitting in with the existing staff. Your reader should be able to envision pasting this headshot and bio right onto their website staff page.

Ask for Résumé Review

Draft a résumé according to the points above, then share it with your mentorship team for their input. Consider also showing it to someone unfamiliar with the world of yoga, and listen carefully to their feedback and questions.

At yogateacherhandbook.com, you'll find a few sample résumés and a template for creating your own.

ASSETS

Your biography and résumé will help you land jobs, which we'll discuss in the next chapter. Condensed elements of your bio and résumé will appear in your marketing material, so they are a great place to start. For your ongoing promotion, you'll need to collect a few more assets. These are the materials that will appear in your marketing, whether it's in print or online. They should at the very least include a photo or two, a few lines about your offerings (classes, workshops, retreats), and a consistent look: a particular typeface and color palette that you use throughout your marketing materials (yep, that's your *brand*).

Photos

At least every other year during your yoga teaching career, you should spend the time and money to secure high-quality photos from a professional photographer or a talented amateur with nice equipment. Hairstyles, fashion, and bodies change over the years, as will your yoga practice. Having and using current photos will provide an up-to-date picture of what you, your practice, and your class look like. This will help you connect best with the right students for what you offer.

For your session, create a shot list of images you want to be sure to get. A good photographer will have some suggestions, but when you are both operating from a list of must-have shots, things will go most smoothly. Start with headshots, perhaps with a few different looks: one in a yoga top, one in street clothes, one with a big, natural smile, one more posed or artistic.

You'll also want images of you in a variety of asanas. Be sure that many of these are accessible poses (think tree, not bird of paradise) where your face, smiling or with a pleasantly neutral expression, is visible. While forward folds can feel great to do, in general they don't photograph well for marketing purposes. Choose instead standing poses that you know virtually all of your students can do with ease.

If you have an advanced asana practice or want to shoot more artistic images, have fun, but save these pictures for promoting an advanced-pose workshop or using on social media with a caption putting them in context.

It's also smart to have photos of you teaching a class. Every person who's photographed must explicitly agree to the use of their likeness, so it's smartest to gather a small group of your peers—for example, your colleagues from yoga teacher training—and stage a class. You'll also get more experienced yogis that way, with prettier form. You can do a round robin, with each of you teaching over the course of an hour, and you can pool the cost of the photographer. Everyone will wind up with photos to use for promotion. Or you can choose a few regular students who are familiar with your sequences and cues. When potential students look at your photos, they should be able to project themselves into the frame and envision taking your class.

If there will be a photographer in a regular class for some reason, like a local media outlet doing a story on the studio, be sure to get all the students' explicit agreement to be photographed. To be safe, you can create or download a photo waiver (aka model release form) to have students sign. You'll find one at yogateacherhandbook.com.

Think about the background in your photos and choose something evergreen. Don't use an easily-identified studio for marketing pictures, then promote your classes in other studios in the same market using the space. That's confusing to students, as it muddles the clarity of the studio's brand and yours.

Look for a neutral background: Choose a familiar outdoor space, or use a white background. If you don't have access to a studio with a plain white wall, most professional photographers will have a white paper roll or scrim to use as a backdrop. If you expect to record video in a set at home, take some photos there. Or, if your hometown has notable architecture, geographical fixtures, or public art (the beach, Gateway Arch, Chicago Bean), take some pictures there. They will be evergreen, provided you still keep that town as your home base.

Put Down the Camera Phone

Please do not take photos yourself while you are teaching your class, especially while your students are in savasana or in happy baby! That's trespassing on their privacy and violating the safe space you've created during class. It's also not aesthetically pleasing when the room is appropriately dark. If you want a good savasana picture, put it on your shot list for your next photo shoot, and get a photo of you smiling while offering an assist to a student who has signed a photo waiver.

Graphics

Choose a color palette and font that convey your brand. If you teach exciting power classes, you might want to choose a bright color and a strong typeface; if you specialize in gentle and restorative yoga, perhaps a more muted palette and more delicate script are in order. If you're not sure which direction to go, assemble a mood board of sites and graphics that you like, and once you've collected several, you'll likely see a common theme emerging.

A graphic designer can help—perhaps you'll find one who will trade advice for yoga. You can also commission design help online at Fiverr and set your own price point. If you are making your own design decisions, choose a font that is widely available, like the fonts you'll find in the Microsoft suite or the Google free fonts. It will make it simple to pass the work to a designer down the road.

While you may have a bunch of energy and excitement around developing a brand as a yoga teacher, you probably don't need a logo per se. If you feel you simply must have one, seek a graphic designer who will work on trade.

WEBSITE

You don't need a fancy website. Even a single page with a smiling photo, your schedule, a brief bio, and your contact information will suffice.

In order to do this, you need a URL—universal resource locator—which is your address on the web. If you don't already own yourname.com, please put this book down and try to buy it now! While you're at it, consider buying yogawithyourname.com, yournameyoga.com, yournameyogayourstate.com, and yourname.yoga (yes, .yoga is now a domain you can register). You can do this at any domain registry service like Go Daddy, Google Domains, or Web.com. If you have ideas for businesses, like a dream of owning a yoga studio or writing an ebook that you would sell on a website, buy domain names for those projects at the same time. Rates go down substantially when you buy in bulk.

Owning a URL is like having rights to a street address. Next, you need to put a house at that address, and there are a few ways to do that. One is to go with an all-in-one web builder, like Squarespace or 1and1.com. You can even use these services to buy your URL. They will offer a variety of templates—like house designs—that you can customize to align with your brand. They will even host your site. Your web host is like the lot where the house is built. This is a good place to start, like buying a starter home. As you choose between services, think of your medium- and long-term goals. If you intend to add video content or offer class or workshop registration through your site, you may find an outfit that easily supports these features.

If, down the road, you have specific needs or a big budget, you can get a custom-designed website like what you'll see at carolinayogacompany.com or sagerountree.com. In this house analogy, these are architect-designed sites. A graphic designer and a web developer work together on them like an architect and a contractor, or a design/builder and an interior designer.

A good starter website for a professional yoga teacher will include the following elements. They can be sections of a single page or discrete pages, but it should be very clear to the viewer how to navigate between these elements.

Welcome

Open with a warm, enthusiastic sentence of welcome, ideally accompanied by an image of you in an accessible yoga pose, smiling at the camera (not a back shot), and possibly also a smiling headshot.

This should say to the viewer, either implicitly or explicitly: "You will find a sense of connection and joy in classes with Chris," or whatever your message is. What will your viewer gain by taking your class? How will they feel? Mellow? Stronger? Challenged? Uplifted? All of the above?

About

It's time to deploy the bio you've already started! Condense it to a paragraph or two about your yoga journey, again, with a focus on how your students will feel once they connect with you.

Schedule

Keep an updated schedule of where you teach, when, how much it costs, where students can sign up, and where they should park/how to get there via public transit. Add full class descriptions to set students' expectations. Set yourself a reminder to update this frequently, about every three months. If you offer workshops, series, or retreats, feature them here.

If you offer private lessons, include a description, along with a price list and a way to book. Depending on the web platform you're using, there may be appointment scheduling built in; you can also use your calendar software to assign availability, or invite your students to contact you to schedule a lesson.

Thus, depending on your teaching offerings, your schedule page could have sections or separate pages called "Find a Class," "Take a Workshop," "Go on Retreat," "Schedule a Private Lesson," and so on. Note that each of these is a call to action focused on the reader.

Contact

Give students a way to reach you with any questions. If you don't want to post your email address, there are some workarounds. One is to create a new address (yournameyoga@gmail.com, or info@yournameyoga.com, once you learn how to deploy the custom email addresses that come when you buy a URL), which you can use as a stand-alone or forward to your main account. Another is to use a contact form, which your web builder would supply.

Similarly, if you don't want to give out your private phone number, you can create a Google Voice number. Any calls or texts to that number can be forwarded to your private number.

Art

Each of these pages or sections should be illustrated with a high-quality photo. Unless you explicitly teach advanced asana, make these accessible poses. Be sure your face is visible in at least two-thirds of these shots. A shot from behind can be artful, but having too many on your site makes you look shy.

If you have some artistic photographs of you in more difficult poses, list them in a section or on a page called "Gallery," and consider adding a blurb about how long it took you to learn these moves and whether they appear in your regular class. Be sure to credit your photographer. If they are open to bookings, link to their site.

Other Elements

Video. Nice, but not critical to have unless you offer video content online, is a short snippet of you teaching. This could be either a video shot in a staged class where all of the students know they are being filmed, or a quick lesson on a single pose or a unique way to use a prop. A minute or two of video footage goes a really long way at conveying your energy as a teacher, and it will be useful both to potential students and to prospective employers. We will cover how to produce such videos in chapters 7 and 10.

Music. If you use music in class, you can link your playlists on your website. Be sure that you have paid attention to appropriate licensing fees, which we discuss in part 3.

Testimonials. It's nice to have a blurb or two from your mentors and your students about your teaching. If you're citing a mentor, use their full name and, if it's helpful, a positioning phrase "Sage Rountree, co-owner of the Carolina Yoga Company and author of *The Athlete's Guide to Yoga.*" If you're citing a student, a first name is probably enough.

Booking details. If you intend to offer workshops as a traveling teacher, it is helpful to prepare a workshop offerings document. This will be unpacked in part 4. Your offerings list could go on a page called "Bookings" on your website, or you can simply invite people to contact you to request the document.

MEDIA KIT

Since you'll already have collected these assets for your website, you can arrange them all in a folder as a media kit. This can be passed to any studios that host a workshop, as well as to journalists who interview you as an expert. I keep mine in Dropbox and share the folder whenever it is requested. Your media kit should include:

- ▶ Bios in various lengths, including one around 50 words, one around 150 to 200 words, and one full-length biography; when you are presenting a lecture or workshop, these are invaluable for the people tasked with introducing you.
- ▶ Headshots: recent professional photos of you smiling at the camera; one or two well-lit, high-resolution pictures are plenty.

▶ Action shots: photos of you teaching students who know they are being photographed (obtain a model release!); if appropriate for your brand and workshop content, include photos of you in asanas related to the workshop.
▶ Book covers, podcast cover images, logos, or other supporting materials.

Update your media kit regularly.

Self-Promotion as Service

If promotion—specifically self-promotion—feels icky to you, try to recast your thinking about it as shining your light. You can't help people when you hide your light under a bushel. Promotion is easy when you know exactly who you are and how you can help people using the skills you've developed. Then it feels less like selling and more like service. When you have a clear message of who you are and how you can help, you'll naturally draw the right students to you and organically help raise the tide of yoga. This rising tide lifts all boats, so your mindful presentation of yourself and yoga's benefits will naturally also help your colleagues and the field in general.

NEWSLETTERS

Real talk: Setting up and sending newsletters is one of my least favorite tasks. But it's one that, done right, will keep your students invested in your offerings and ensure your workshops and retreats are successful. Like many tedious chores, it feels easier if you spend a few minutes a week tending to it and an hour or two a month batching all your other efforts on it: collecting assets, writing copy, scheduling your content.

Permission-Based Marketing

The formal term for your email newsletter is "permission-based marketing." *Permission* is the critical word here: Your students need to opt in to receiving your email newsletter. You can't just take student addresses from your sign-ups—or, worse, from your studio's scheduling software—and add them to your list. Students must give you permission to send them emails.

How to get permission varies on where you are teaching and what the venue's policies are. When you are at a gym, studio, or anywhere you are not the clear boss, be very sure about whether you can solicit addresses from students. Once you have explicit permission from the venue, there are a few options. If you are having students sign a waiver, you can add a yes/no box to the waiver form. Or you can have a separate clipboard for students to add email addresses, which you'll then manually input. If you're savvy, you could have your webpage open on a laptop or tablet and let students subscribe themselves. Try to capture them while they're present; an offhand mention like "You can sign up for my newsletter at mywebsite.com" isn't going to gain you many subscribers.

That said, your website is a natural place to invite viewers to become subscribers. Do this via a pop-up form or a form that is always visible in the sidebar or footer. Offer something of value in exchange for signing up. I offer a code for a premium video, which gives recipients a 48-hour rental of one of my Core Strength for Real People episodes. You might offer a pose explanation, a favorite yoga sequence, a playlist, a recording of a guided meditation, or a coupon code for your next workshop or series.

It needs to be very obvious for subscribers how they can quickly unsubscribe themselves from your newsletter. You can't simply BCC your list and not say "reply with 'unsubscribe' if you would rather stop receiving these." (And don't *ever* simply CC your list with email addresses visible, which is a violation of privacy.) Readers need to be able to get out easily. This is one of many reasons to choose a respected platform for sending your newsletter. These platforms will also save you the work of removing people from a list manually, and, if you toggle the right setting, will save you the pain of seeing who unsubscribes from your list.

Choose a Platform

You're likely familiar with the big players in the business: Constant Contact, iContact, MailChimp. There is even a yoga-specific newsletter software, Namaste Light. Each of these offers scaled pricing, so when your list is small they are low-cost or even free. As your list grows, so does your monthly fee.

For several years, I've been using a Wordpress plug-in called MailPoet. It's housed on my website, which is based in Wordpress, and it allows both for creation of newsletters from scratch and for posts to the blog on my site to go out as newsletters. This suits my desire to spend as little time as possible on my newsletter: When I have something to share, I put it in a blog post, which then gets disseminated via various channels: the blog itself, the RSS feed that readers can subscribe to, my social media (via the Jetpack plugin), and, every Tuesday when there is fresh content, my newsletter. This does mean my newsletter isn't distributed on a regular once-a-month schedule, but it also means the newsletter goes out only when there is relevant content.

Each of these platforms will allow you to segment your audience so that you can subdivide your list to send the most useful messaging to each discrete user. You could set up a campaign welcoming new subscribers, so that they receive a few weeks of introduction to you and your work. You can denote some subscribers as festivalgoers or potential retreat-goers or athletes or yoga teachers, whatever segments work for your base.

Write and Batch Your Work

No newsletter needs to be very long. Shorter is better. Your readers will likely look at only the first screen or so of the message, so don't bury your lede. A line or two about an upcoming offering, a link to a longer blog post about your theme for the month, or even a share of something you found meaningful is all you need. Give your readers a clear call to action, like a button or a link saying "Sign up here!" or "Download the meditation." A rule of thumb: Your newsletter should effectively be no longer than three social media posts. Two is better, and one is often enough, especially if it's for a big announcement like a retreat or a forthcoming book.

Don't overlook the title and the secondary line, which is what displays in readers' email applications as a preview of the content. These should match your teaching tone and invite the reader to open the email itself. Instead of "November News," go with something like "Ready to Run Away to Costa Rica?" or "You'll Doze Right Off with This Meditation for Better Sleep." Survey the offerings from both local and national teachers and pinpoint what you think works well, then model your newsletters on that formula.

If you feel, as I do, that setting up your newsletters is like pulling teeth, block out a few hours, set up in your favorite working environment, and knock out several at once. Any newsletter service will allow you to schedule these in advance.

Aim to send a newsletter at least quarterly, so that your readers remember who you are. But, at the other end of the spectrum, don't send newsletters more than once a week unless you do it rarely, in service of a special event.

Strategize Your Newsletter

Any task is less daunting once you start to break it down into smaller chunks. Here's how to get started on creating a newsletter.

▶ Subscribe to several teachers' newsletters to have role models. Choose peers in your area and some nationally or internationally known teachers.

▶ List the steps you will take to get sign-ups and what you'll need to do to implement them (e.g., speak to the manager at the venue where you teach).

▶ Look at the available options—one might be via the website builder you choose—and settle on a newsletter service. Read that service's best-practices articles, and if they offer a video series or a help session to get you up to speed, use it.

▶ List some content you can promote. This could be a video series you've created, or a blog post you have written, or the handout from a workshop you've taught. All of these will be explained in part 4. You can also point to someone else's content that you found especially helpful.

▶ Write a plan to "drip" (trickle out piece by piece) this content across several weeks or months of newsletters.

▶ Draft your first newsletter. Each service will have a set of templates for you to choose from. Find the one that is most in line with your brand, pop in your content, and schedule it.

▶ Check your statistics. What was clicked on? Let that guide you to your next newsletter topic.

SOCIAL MEDIA

Social media is a major tool for yoga teachers to reach their current and potential students and to develop their brand. There are millions of directions to go with your social media and other content campaigns—and the social media landscape is constantly changing, so you'll need to adapt accordingly. But here's how to get started with social media, or to revamp your approach to make it more systematic and professional.

Find Role Models

Start by considering your current and your desired student base, which may be the same or could be quite different. Are they using social media, and if so, what platform will you find them on most of the time? If your students don't use social media, you may not want to put much time or energy into establishing a presence there. There's no requirement that teachers use social media! If a particular platform confuses you or makes you feel anxious and irritated every time you use it, don't waste effort in establishing a foothold there. Better yet, consider deleting the app from your phone or even suspending your account. Instead, enhance your presence in the places you *do* enjoy scrolling, commenting, and posting. It will be a much more positive experience.

If you do enjoy spending time on social media, you likely follow several yoga teachers already. Think about why you chose to follow them and how you respond to their posts. Make note of the teachers whose message resonates best with you—and those whose promotion doesn't work for you. From your reactions, you can reverse engineer a strategy of your own that feels authentic to you.

Some of my favorites on Instagram are, for students, Mary Ochsner (@maryochsner), and for teachers, Jenni Rawlings (@jenni_rawlings). Mary's work gives bite-size tidbits for people to add yoga to their lives at any stage. Jenni consistently posts creative exercise physiology–based sequences that could fit into the context of any flow class to keep it challenging and varied. Both women deliver high-quality content on a regular schedule. Follow them for inspiration—and to recognize how much work this truly is!

Consider Establishing a New Business Account

Depending on when you first joined various social networks, your personal page may have evolved into a yoga-business page. Or you may already have a separate account for your yoga business. If you don't, consider creating one now. That will both serve your old friends in your hometown who don't want to hear about your upcoming workshops in your new location and help your yoga students see you as a professional. The handle for this account could be @yournameyoga or @yogawithyourname. Take a month or two to post weekly, inviting your yoga students who follow your personal account to follow you there instead. Then you can mention it only every other month or once a quarter, maybe when you post yoga-related content to your personal page: "For more yoga content, please follow my business account at @yournameyoga."

Depending on the platform, this new account can be set up as a business account, rather than a personal account. On Instagram, for example, this gives you access to "Insights," statistics on how many people are viewing your posts, saving them, and clicking through to your profile, as well as a few demographics about who these viewers are (age, gender, region). Looking at these metrics will show you what content is most popular with your followers, and you can then create more along those lines. And if you want to be sponsored by a brand, the brand may want to see your statistics to determine your reach.

Create a Content Calendar

While you may have been posting on social media on an ad hoc basis—when you feel like you have something to say—you can and should plan your posts just as you do for your newsletter. Develop a content calendar with your upcoming events, like the addition of a new class, a workshop, a video series, or a retreat. Work back from the event date to schedule posts promoting the event. These posts can mention a problem that students may have and how your event will solve it.

Your content calendar could be in a spreadsheet, or, for a minor fee, you can schedule your content using software like Hootsuite or Buffly. These applications will post your content for you on a schedule of your choice, or they will suggest the best time to post automatically. This can be nice if you like to batch your work for maximum efficiency. Be sure to visit the posts once they are up and answer any student questions or thank them for their comments.

PRINT MARKETING

While you probably don't need many printed materials, it's good to have a few. You can design and order these yourself online using tools like Canva or Moo.

Business Card

Have your name, web address, and professional contact information, including your business social media handles, if you use them. You don't need 500 or 1,000 cards—your information will likely change before you get through that many. Just order 250 and share them liberally.

Postcards

If you are promoting a series or retreat, or a workshop you would really like to fill, consider printing postcards to advertise it. These aren't actual postcards that you would mail—be sure to use all the space on both sides.

Flyers

For workshops, series, and retreats, a single-page flyer can be useful. Before investing much effort in designing and printing these, think through where you might hang them. Use big fonts and bright colors, which makes the flyer more accessible to any reader. Less is more. Be sure your flyer covers the basics of what, when, and where, and that it's obvious where to register.

ADVERTISING

The aphorism attributed to John Wanamaker goes, "Half the money I spend advertising is wasted; the trouble is I don't know which half." That was especially true in the era of print advertising, where it was very difficult to track whether and which advertising worked. Print advertising is out of virtually every teacher's budget, and you'll get better, more trackable results by instead focusing on online ads. These can be on Google Adwords or on social media like Facebook or Instagram. If you are generating good content, which you'll be equipped to do when you finish this book, you won't need to advertise much to garner awareness of your brand as a teacher. Advertising may be useful when you have something specific to promote, like workshops, retreats, and online content, which which we cover in part 4. With online ads, you can dial in the audience so that your ads are targeted to the people most likely to be interested in how you can help them with yoga.

PROMOTION IN CLASS

Depending on where you are teaching, you may have a clipboard of studio announcements to read before class. Perhaps you can add to this a mention of your own offerings, especially at the studio itself. If you do this, be sure not to overdo it. Mention one thing at the start of class and reiterate it briefly again at the end, rather than subjecting students to a litany of sales pitches. If you've got the go-ahead to point students to your newsletter or website, let them know where they can find more information and sign up.

Be very clear on the studio guidelines before mentioning anything you are offering off-site. Some studios disallow *any* promotion for outside events, even a mention of your social media or newsletter, regarding that as solicitation of the studio's students. You may even see a nonsolicitation clause in your contract to this effect. Others, like ours at Carolina Yoga Company, allow you to promote outside events like retreats, but only orally during your class. All paper you bring, like a postcard touting your event, leaves with you. Otherwise, the counter and flyer boards are riddled with conflicting branding and we wind up devoting all our marketing space to something we don't make money on. But this policy is unusual; expect the first instead, and be sure to ask your hiring manager so that you are completely clear on what your studio expects from you. Good communication will prevent suffering on all sides.

Are you pumped? I hope so! Of course, you need an offering to promote, so let's talk about how to get your first class or make a move into a new student base by creating opportunities to teach a regular weekly class.

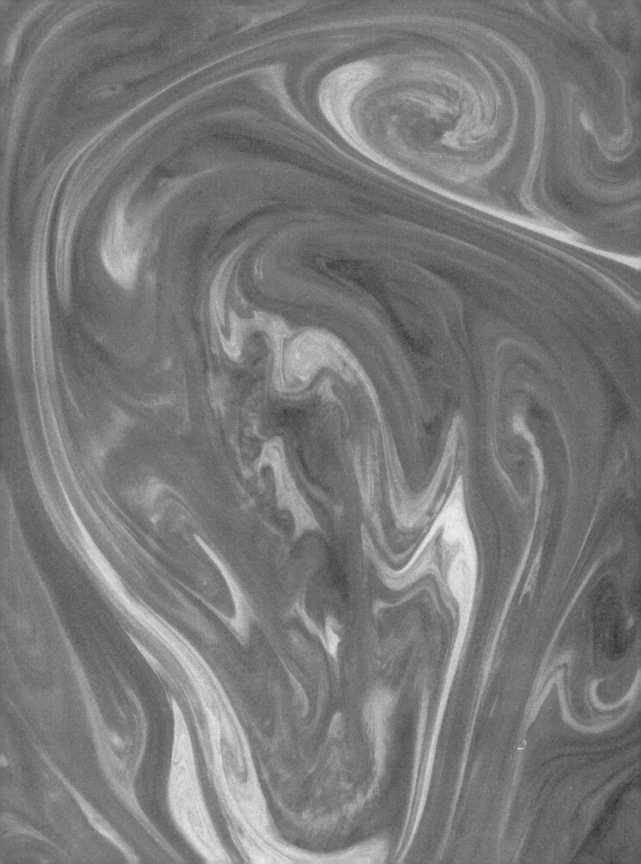

5

Getting a Regular Class Gig

· ·

YOU PICKED UP THIS BOOK either because you are a prospective or new teacher just getting your start, or because you've been teaching for a while and are eager to take your career to the next level. Either way, you are likely ready to secure new teaching slots. Here's how to get started—in person or online.

GYM

A gym is a typical first landing spot for students fresh out of teacher training, and it's a good starter gig. There's a built-in membership of students, which means you'll get plenty of people in class with a wide range of bodies and ages. This is a wonderful way to hone your teaching skills.

Approaching the Gym

Start by taking a look at the website to see if there are instructions on how to apply. If not, drop in and ask at the desk. While you're at it, see if there is a day pass rate or some other way for you to spend some time in the facility, and ideally to take at least one class. Ask who programs group fitness and the best way to contact them. Meet them in person if you can, introduce yourself, and if they are amenable, get their contact information so you can follow up with a résumé and cover letter.

If you can't meet in person, send an email with a paragraph introducing yourself, detailing briefly your experience and availability, and offer to come by in person for an interview at the programmer's convenience. If you get such an interview, arrive early with a big smile, and offer to give an audition, which we'll discuss in a moment.

Payment

Typical payment per class at a gym can range from $15 to $45. An added perk is free gym access, which can be worth $100 or more each month. This is especially useful if there is free child care and you have a young kid—your child can be cared for while you teach or work out. And free membership can give you a chance to take other group exercise classes, as many of the fundamental skills of a good movement teacher carry across disciplines. You might find that your time in a Pilates, cycling, or weightlifting class elevates your awareness of classroom management, good pedagogy, clear cuing, kinesiology, and anatomy in ways that directly improve your abilities as a yoga teacher.

Most places—gyms, studios, corporate gigs—pay an hourly rate per class. This could be $15 to $45 or more at a gym or studio, and might be $85 or more for a corporate class that brings a teacher into the office. At Carolina Yoga Company, we use a different, less common model, $x/head. This rewards teachers who work to attract and retain students, as teacher pay increases with class size. Depending on experience, x may be anything from $5 to $6.50. We pay 70 percent for series and workshops. But most gyms and studios pay by the hour. We will explore money in great detail later, as well as how you might eventually grow your part-time job as a yoga teacher into a full-time profession.

Professional Modes of Contact

Whenever possible, speak to your potential hiring manager in person. Dress professionally: Business casual would never be wrong in the yoga field. If you wear yoga clothes, add an overlayer that covers your bottom so you don't show up clad completely in skintight items. Present yourself as you would to a student: Be warm, friendly, approachable, confident, and authoritative.

If you cannot be present in person, send an email that you have carefully proofread. Keep your language relatively formal and use the same punctuation you would in a printed letter, not a text. If you have your yoga website ready, include a link under your name or as part of your signature file.

If your email goes unanswered, follow up with a phone call. Leaving voice mail is OK as a last resort, but emails are more likely to be answered, as there is a tangible, visible presence of them in your recipient's inbox.

Unless you are explicitly cued to do so, do not use social media direct messages like Facebook Messenger for your professional communications, especially around hiring. These are tough to keep track of and easy to ignore, and they require your correspondent to take at least one extra step every time they want to reply to you.

STUDIOS

Approaching the Studio

Go to the studio. Teaching yoga is a public-facing job—see how it appears to the public at the places you would like to teach. Applying for a teaching slot is not like applying for an office job, where it would be odd to show up and spend time in a cubicle to get the vibe of the place before sending a résumé and cover letter.

That you should start by visiting the studio should be patently obvious, but we regularly get queries about teaching positions from people fresh out of some other studio's teacher training who have never been to our studio. These naive applicants get a stock answer from us:

> We have an overabundance of teachers right now, both on our schedule and on our sub list. When we do hire, we like to choose from among the folks who have been practicing at the studio regularly. If you're interested in teaching at Carolina Yoga Company, that's a great place to start, so that we can get to know each other and so that you can understand the studio culture and student needs. We definitely extend our student/teacher class rate to yoga teachers!

To avoid being the recipient of such a brush-off, be sure to go to the studio. Sign up for their intro offer and go to several classes. This not only shows the hiring manager that you are earnest but also gives you a chance to be sure this studio is a good fit for your teaching. It may not be, so doing your due diligence is critical. Ask students about their experience and their suggestions of classes and teachers. Take a broad sampling of the studio's offerings, which will position you well to talk about them with authority.

Speak to the teachers after class. Pay them an honest compliment about something you especially liked in class. Tell them you are interested in joining the staff. Ask how frequently the schedule changes and who is in charge of writing it. And after you have made several visits, approach that person with a humble introduction and enthusiastic offer to audition. This ideally would happen face-to-face, at a moment when the hiring director is not busy. If that's tough to manage, write a kind, clear, error-free email. Either way, your message should hit these points:

▶ You've had a positive experience at the studio, with reference to the classes/teachers you've enjoyed and what made them memorable

▶ You are a new/experienced teacher interested in teaching there. If you have a specialty or special interest—yin yoga, prenatal yoga, kids yoga, yoga for healthy aging, *yoga en español*—mention it! If your schedule is especially open, or you love early-morning or late-evening classes, mention that.

▶ You are a graduate of X training program and its lead teacher is happy to give you a reference. (Of course, confirm this by asking your teacher trainer first; you may have already done this when you constructed your résumé.)

▶ If applicable: You have studied from or learned alongside a particular teacher already on the studio staff.

▶ Since your graduation, you have led classes to Y students in Z locations.

▶ You are eager to offer an audition and to sub a class or guest teach a portion of class to give them a sense of your teaching style.

▶ If applicable: You are familiar with the business side of MindBody software, if the studio uses it, or other relevant platforms.

Include your résumé and a link to your website, where the hiring manager will find a smiling picture of you and a short bio. These don't belong in the email, which should be as short as possible while covering the above points.

If you don't get a response, follow up in two weeks or so, then again in two months. Timing is everything. At Carolina Yoga, for example, our schedules are written quarterly. Someone who approaches us just before the new scheduling period opens is more likely to get our attention than someone who catches us right after the new schedule begins. Ask when schedules are set, and present a reminder of your enthusiasm just before that period.

Staying Positive

As happens at the entry level of many professions, in yoga teaching, you may hit a catch-22: You need experience to teach, but you need to get in to gain experience. With an eye to your bottom line, you may be able to say yes to less-than-optimal time slots to get your foot in the door. Sometimes those become your favorite slots because of the students.

While you may have your heart set on a studio position, sometimes gaining experience elsewhere is the real ticket in. Look at the wide range of places where you could be helping students: in gyms, at community centers, in nursing homes. Teaching wherever you can will refine your teaching skills, serve your students, and gain you some experience for when you return to pitch the studio again. You may even find these gigs pay better and reward your soul more!

Payment

There are many different models for payment at yoga studios. While you may not find much wiggle room when you are hired, it's useful to know the models you may encounter.

Some pay a flat fee per class, as you saw in the gym model. This rate may depend on your experience and on your level of training, including any specializations you have, such as prenatal yoga. As at a gym, it may vary from $15 to $45 or higher per class, and some studios offer a no-show payment of $15 or so if no one comes.

Pay rate: $15 no-show, $25 per class
Zero students: $15
Six students: $25
Twelve students: $25
Thirty students: $25
Forty students: $25

Some studios, like ours, pay per head at either a set rate—in our case, up to $6.50 per student—or a percentage of the revenue that the student brings in, such as 50 percent. This has some obvious advantages. The more students you can bring in, the bigger your paycheck. Both the studio and the teacher are invested in attracting students. On the other hand, if no one comes to class, you don't get paid.

Pay rate: $6.50/head
Zero students: $0
Six students: $39
Twelve students: $78
Thirty students: $195
Forty students: $260

Many studios offer a hybrid between the per-class and per-head rates. There is a base rate for a class, and if the class has over a set number of students—say, ten—you're paid a set amount of bonus per student—say, $2. There may also be a maximum, so that you are never paid more than a set amount—say, $65.

Pay rate: $25 base, $2/student bonus for everyone after ten students, cap $65
Zero students: $0
Six students: $25
Twelve students: $29
Thirty students: $65
Forty students: $65

Some studios are run as donation studios. This model can take various forms: It can be on a sliding scale, with a suggested range of money to pay; an invitation to pay what you can; or even a chance to do chores or donate goods in exchange for a class. (Once, visiting Colorado Springs for work at the Olympic Training Center, I brought a copy of my first book to a donation studio there. Another student offered a few heads of broccoli, and the teacher was equally enthusiastic about both.) The concept behind donation studios is very sweet, and it echoes the origins of yoga as a practice where the students supported the teacher. When the donation model mixes with capitalism, though, problems can emerge. I spoke to a teacher who reported that at the donation studio where she taught, her average donation was $4, of which half was to go to the studio for using the space, meaning she was earning $2 per student. And I worry that the students were not valuing the class or her time as they might have if the rate were set at even $10 per class, or an hour of chores in the space.

Keeping Your Job: How to Be Useful

The best teachers contribute to the overall success of the studio or gym. They don't just show up, teach, and leave; they participate in classes as students, and they find ways to make the manager's work easier and the operation run smoothly. You can do this in small ways: Take care to train your students to put props back in order, to fold the blankets in the studio's preferred way, and to be quiet in the hall, if that's needed for sound reasons. When you can, substitute teach to help out your colleagues—this earns you major brownie points with both your peers and your bosses. If you see something that needs doing, do it: Take out the trash, sweep the floor, answer students' questions. If you see something that could improve, let your manager know in a kind way with concrete ideas for how to improve it. All of these will lighten management's load and will make you an invaluable staff member, and your ideas will be remembered when primo slots come open on the schedule or pay raises or bonuses are being handed out.

INTERVIEWS AND AUDITIONS

Depending on the hiring process at your prospective new host business, you may be run through a series of interviews and auditions. Treat your interview as you would any job interview. Do research about the business, take a close look at its current schedule, and see where you could fit in or add value—by adding a class at a time that is currently not used, for example. Prepare questions to ask about the business, and especially about its clientele. Be ready to demonstrate that you are an ideal candidate to serve this student base.

Come prepared with a document listing your skills (like the workshops offering form I describe in chapter 10, but with descriptions of classes) or be eager to describe the various classes you can teach. Some gyms and studios have set sequences or tight parameters around what they offer, in which case they may need to train you. Be careful about committing to lots of expensive training on your dime. Ideally, your employer will train you on the clock or for free as an apprentice.

Some gyms and studios use in-class or faux-class auditions as part of the hiring process. If you are invited to audition, ask smart questions so you can get a clear picture of what is expected of you and how you can succeed. They might include:

▶ Logistics: Note when, where, how long, and whether you should use music, and whether hands-on assists are standard at the studio.

▶ Subject matter: Would your hiring contact like a full class or a segment? If a segment, which segment—the beginning, middle, or end of class? (Sometimes several candidates audition together, each leading a small portion of the class.) What style of yoga would they like to see you teach?

▶ Audience: Who will your students be in the audition? If they are staff or studio owners, should you treat them as new students or as the experienced practitioners they are? If they are students, what level of experience should you expect them to have?

Once you know what to prepare, treat it as a regular class. Think through what you want to teach, how you would expand or contract your teaching if the available time changes, and ways to modify for different bodies and needs. We'll explore how to prepare in depth in part 3.

At the end of your audition, ask for feedback if it is not immediately given. Your auditioners have likely seen many people teach and should have some useful commentary for you, whether or not you are ultimately hired to teach for them. As with any interview, follow up with a thank-you note or email in a day or two, regardless of the outcome. A "no" this time can be a "yes" next time if you make a good impression and work to improve between tries.

ONLINE

Getting Started

As the yoga industry adapts to a changing world, many teachers and studios are migrating online. Not every teacher will want or need to have an online presence, so you should consider whether it's the right move for you. You'll know it's right when you are excited, if a little scared, and eager to share your teaching in platforms beyond face-to-face class-rooms. Breaking into the online world as a brand-new teacher will involve a little ambi-tion, a measure of comfort and agility with the platforms you choose (social media, video, audio), and a healthy dose of self-promotional hustle. Just like with your in-person teach-ing and promotion, it helps to be really clear on who you are, what your message is, why you are teaching, and most importantly, who your audience is and how you can help them with yoga. Getting clear on the answers to those questions will help you decide where and what to teach online, and it will help you craft a marketing message that feels authentic.

Approaching the Host

As a result of social distancing initiatives brought about during the coronavirus pan-demic, many studios began to offer online content alongside in-person classes. This con-tent can be either live streams or recordings of classes at the studio—or a separately cre-ated library of classes and tutorials. While studios' online teachers are often the same as their existing in-person teachers, if you have skill with teaching on video, you may be able to work your way into the rotation. (We will discuss hosting your own online offerings in chapter 10.) If you are just getting started as a teacher, this can be a mutually beneficial relationship. You get to use the studio's equipment, expertise, and platform—and they get the benefit of your teaching.

Start as you would with an in-person class: Get a sense of what is being offered. Watch several different teachers' classes to have a sense of the aesthetic, tone, and energy that the studio puts forth. Is there much demonstration? Is there much back-and-forth with students in live classes? Do students turn off their video cameras or leave them on? Is there music? Do the lessons presume students have their own props, suggest how to make do with things around the house, or go prop-free? How does what you have to offer complement the existing content or fill a niche that is not being served?

Next, approach the hiring manager with an expression of interest—in person, if possible, or online. Detail the classes you've taken, the vibe you've picked up on, and how your own offerings will be a good fit. Send a link to a short clip of your teaching online (don't send the video file itself; these can be too big for email). If the studio offers video recorded only on set in their own space, seek to create a space that echoes the studio brand. If you don't have access to professional-grade equipment, explain what you used to record your sample. Offer to give a full-length audition or interview, as per the practices previously detailed.

Payment

Just as there are a range of payment practices for in-person classes, payment for video classes varies. Some studios will offer only a set fee per live stream or recording. Others offer royalties based on views of the video when it is viewed from the studio library.

Since video classes can be archived in ways that live classes can't be, be clear with the studio about who owns the intellectual property rights to the recording. If you were to leave your association with the host, would your videos still be available on their platform? Would you still be paid? Be clear on the terms, and have a written contract.

Likewise, be clear on whether you are allowed to mention your other content in the videos you create for this platform. Effectively, you're taking the in-person contract and adapting it for the online environment.

DO IT YOURSELF

Outside of the gym or studio, there is a world full of places where you could teach yoga! This includes community centers, church basements, middle-school gymnasiums, martial arts and dance studios, art galleries, hotels, and the great outdoors. Increasingly, it means online in video classes, social media posts, and other formats. If you would like to take a do-it-yourself approach to offering a class, we'll discuss options for setting up alternative classes in chapter 10.

Whether you are looking for a regular class gig or already have one, it's important to make sure you're prepared when it comes to money. A little knowledge will serve you well as you agree—or even negotiate—to take on your first class. Not all of us have this knowledge up front! As I moved from being a very part-time teacher to becoming the owner of several wellness businesses, I had to learn about good business practices around labor law, accounting, and other back-of-the-house issues. Let these lessons I've learned guide you as you talk to professional advisers about how to structure your own business.

EMPLOYEES VERSUS INDEPENDENT CONTRACTORS

In the United States, yoga teachers will be hired in one of two categories: *employees* or *independent contractors*. Employees fill out a W-4 form at hiring and have estimated income tax, Social Security, and Medicare deducted from their paycheck. They receive a W-2 form at the end of the tax year. Full-time employees also may have some rights and benefits, like the ability to file for unemployment, paid vacation time, and, in larger companies, health insurance. Independent contractors fill out a W-9 form at hiring and receive a 1099 form at the end of the year if they earned at least $600 over the year. Payments to independent contractors contain no deductions; it's incumbent on the contractor to track and pay all taxes.

Employees may be told what to do, when they will do it, and exactly how it should be done. Employees are subject to work evaluations, and in general can be far more tightly controlled. Independent contractors are not: They are hired to achieve a task and should be left to their own devices as to how that work is done. A major upside of working as an independent contractor is being able to write off all reasonable business expenses, which we will touch on in a moment.

To teach at a gym, you will likely be hired as an employee. If you create your own classes, you will be a sole proprietor, which functions similarly to an independent contractor. But if you teach at a studio, the situation depends on the individual company's structure. Many studios prefer the ease of classifying teachers as independent contractors, as it cuts down on hiring paperwork, payroll costs, and taxes paid by the studio.

Others are making the shift toward employees. California, for example, has a law requiring studios to treat all teachers as employees rather than independent contractors. You generally won't have a choice between the two. Be clear on what basis you are being hired, and educate yourself about the tax implications.

Either way, be aware of what your paycheck should include. Keep track of your hours worked or number of students taught, and be sure that your paycheck accurately reflects it. There's plenty of room for error in payroll processing, as humans are involved in many steps of the process—and of course the programs themselves can have a glitch. When in doubt, ask!

Invoicing

To follow the letter of the law, independent contractors should submit invoices. If you're not familiar with creating an invoice, you'll find a sample template at yogateacherhandbook.com. Most word processing programs and all bookkeeping programs like QuickBooks and FreshBooks will also generate invoices for you. An invoice should include the date, your name, your address, a line describing the work being billed for, and terms of payment: payment due on receipt, Net 15 (payment expected in 15 days), or Net 30 (payment expected in 30 days). If you are using a program to create invoices and have registered for credit card processing with that program, your invoice might include a "pay here" link.

BANKING AND BOOKKEEPING

The exciting part of securing this new job is that you will be paid! When you receive your paycheck, you need to think carefully about where it goes. First, know what your status is: an employee or an independent contractor. If you are an employee, the money from your paycheck can go right into your personal bank account; you might be wise to save a little extra for taxes, but most of your taxes will have been deducted. At the end of the year, your US-based employer will send you a W-2 form for your taxes.

When you are an independent contractor, your paycheck should go into a separate business bank account. Most banks will offer you free checking and savings accounts.

When your paycheck arrives, shunt 30 to 50 percent (or whatever your accountant recommends) into savings to cover your tax burden and save you from a tax-day shock. The rest can be used for your equipment, continuing education, and other legitimate expenses. When you draw from your business checking to give yourself pocket money or cover non-yoga expenses, you'll record this. These are your *distributions*: your net earnings. At the end of the year, your business clients (they aren't technically employers when you aren't an employee) who paid you at least $600 for the year should send you a 1099 form.

Beyond simply depositing money into the bank and using your debit card or checks to pay your expenses, you'll need to track your income and your expenses. This is *bookkeeping*. This could be something you do yourself in software like QuickBooks or Fresh-Books. If you're really busy, you can pay a bookkeeper. Having orderly books means you can quickly see how much you are earning from month to month, which reduces surprises and makes tax reporting simpler.

Since none of us are born knowing how to keep books or estimate taxes, it's worth paying a professional for help. You should start as you mean to go on: The sooner you establish good systems in compliance with the law, the easier it will be to scale as your work increases. Even if you're getting only a few hundred dollars a month from your independent contracting, you should be developing clear bookkeeping systems that can scale up as your yoga business grows. If you haven't worked with an accountant before, it's worth investing some of your yoga earnings to buy an hour of consultation. You might be able to find some free consulting: Some municipalities, counties, and states offer free or reduced-rate advice to sole proprietors or small-business owners. Paying for accounting advice is itself a business expense.

When you are an independent contractor, you can deduct from your taxes legitimate business expenses. Your adviser will help you understand what counts as a business expense. These include supplies like yoga mats and other props, as well as any equipment, including a computer or cell phone, that you use for your business. Your website and any services you use to deliver online content are business expenses. Sadly, you cannot write off your yoga clothes as a "uniform"—that category is for things like mechanic's jumpsuits that you would wear only for work and not for recreation. Continuing education classes—trainings, workshops, even regular classes—and out-of-town travel for continuing education can be deducted. Travel for teaching can probably not be deducted. You will do best to find an accountant who's used to working with small-business owners and sole proprietors, and ask their advice.

Knowing what you really earn from your teaching will help you make smart choices about which jobs to pursue and which offers to take, as well as how much you can spend on operating expenses and professional development.

Payment Processing

When you work directly with clients, you'll need to give them options to pay. This could be by cash or check, of course, but it's nice for your clients to use a credit card (and earn points). There are many services that will handle payment processing for you—while taking a cut, naturally. I use Stripe, which is integrated on my website for people buying courses and books from me, and which also has an app so I can run credit cards in person. You can also look at Square or PayPal, among others, for payment processing. These services will deposit the proceeds from your sale directly into your business bank account, but you'll also want to track them as part of your bookkeeping.

Teachers who offer video content online sometimes ask for payment by donation. This is a tricky term: Is the payment a personal gift (consumer to consumer), or is it payment for services rendered (consumer to business)? Or is it an actual donation to a charity (in which case calling it "donation" is accurate)? To further complicate things, teachers ask for these donations via Venmo or Apple Cash or PayPal as consumer-to-consumer gifts; none of these platforms are technically designed for consumer-to-business payments. To avoid getting in sticky situations with nasty tax implications, I suggest that you charge a fair fee for videos and run your payment processing through merchant services like Stripe or Square. If you want to give a range of price choices, call it "sliding scale" rather than donation. Talk to your accountant to be sure you are fully aware of the implications for your taxes.

SOLE PROPRIETORSHIP VERSUS INCORPORATING

In my own journey as a teacher, I have moved from sole proprietorship to being a share-holder in several different corporations. I've had to learn along the way, with help from professional accountants and attorneys. As a solo teacher, whether you are hosting your own classes and private lessons or working as an independent contractor for several studios, you will file taxes initially as a sole proprietor. These taxes will not be taken out of the paychecks you receive as an independent contractor, so it is critical that you set aside one third to one half of what you take in from your teaching to cover your quarterly tax burden.

When you are making more than five figures a year from your teaching, or if you have plans to hire people to work for you as assistants or teachers in a space you manage, you'll probably want to form a corporation. This is a legal entity that holds your business operations. In the United States, it has its own tax identification number called an EIN, for employer identification number, rather than the Social Security number that is tied to you as an individual.

If you choose to incorporate in the United States, talk to a professional, who will outline the choice between forming an LLC (limited liability company) or an S-Corp (S Corporation, which usually has the designation Inc. after its name). LLCs do not have to pay payroll; S-Corps generally do. If you expect to hire employees down the line, S-Corp may be a wiser choice; if you intend to stay a solo venture, LLC may work for you.

At this stage, you should stop taking your cues from my experience and instead spend the money to talk to a lawyer, who can help you form the corporation, and an accountant, who will explain your tax liability and can prepare your quarterly and annual tax forms. If you're not yet making enough to afford to pay such professionals from your teaching, there's your answer: Incorporation can wait.

LIABILITY

There are several steps that you should take to manage your liability in the event that a student is hurt in your class and sues. These are sometimes called "veils of liability," each of them a curtain between a litigant and your assets. A good attorney will quickly pierce these veils, but that doesn't mean they can be neglected.

Teach Well, Communicate Clearly

The most important self-defense is to cue a safe class and to encourage students to make smart choices at every stage. Several studies have shown that doctors who communicate clearly and cultivate a positive bedside manner are less prone to receiving malpractice lawsuits. Spending some time reminding students to listen to their bodies while also explaining why you are cuing a pose and how to move into and out of it safely is always smart professional practice. We'll discuss safe teaching practices in part 3.

Waivers and Disclaimers

Any student you come into contact with, in a gym or studio class, in a class you host, in a group you visit, or in a private lesson, should sign a waiver and release of indemnification acknowledging that they are taking care of themselves in the class and waiving their right to sue you. This should be signed on paper or electronically at the original contact with the student, then filed somewhere safe for your reference. Since state and national laws vary, it's worth running your waiver draft past a lawyer. Meanwhile, something is better than nothing, so don't hesitate to use the boilerplate waiver you'll find at yogateacher-handbook.com.

For online offerings, include a disclaimer, indicating that viewers practice at their own risk. This can be accomplished through text on the website hosting your videos as well as a quick title card you insert before any video. Run this past your attorney and your insurance agent.

Insurance

While any facility that hires you will have its own liability insurance, that insurance is to cover *their* obligation of liability, not yours. In the event of a suit, the venue's insurance company can be quick to cast the blame on you. You must therefore carry your own liability insurance.

While generally shopping around is a smart plan when buying insurance, in the case of yoga teaching liability insurance, you will find the best deal when you go with the guild and buy either via Yoga Alliance (which uses Alliant for coverage) or Yoga Journal (which uses the Philadelphia). Either of these costs less than $200 per year for tens of thousands of dollars of coverage. Research both and decide which suits your needs. If you are teaching online, talk to the provider about coverage.

Some venues, festivals, and retreat centers will ask you for proof of insurance, and some will ask that you provide a document from your insurer listing the venue as an additional insured location. This is (somewhat) easy to do on your insurance company webpage—you'll navigate to document production, input the venue's name and address, and generate a PDF. If you find it isn't so easy, call the insurer.

Incorporation and Separate Accounts

If you have incorporated as an LLC or S-Corp, you will have an additional veil of liability: A suit would, in theory, go against you as the manager or president of the corporation, and hold against its assets, not against you as an individual with personal bank accounts, a home, a car, and so on. The corporation is sued, not you. This is another reason to keep your yoga income in a separate account under the name of the business. In order for this to work, you need to clearly respect the distinction between your business and personal assets and avoid commingling them. An accountant can help you understand how to do this cleanly. Again, canny lawyers may be able to punch through these veils, but they are useful to have.

Are you still awake? I realize that very little of this is sexy, but it's critical that you think through how to protect your assets and your livelihood. Let it remind you to teach responsibly and to empower your students to make smart choices about their bodies and their movements.

Prepare Your To-Do List

If you do not already have these items in place, write yourself a timeline for getting them as soon as possible, with the next step or steps for each of them.

Accounting

▶ Open business checking and savings accounts.

▶ Find an accountant and prepare a list of questions to ask.

▶ Understand your tax liabilities.

▶ Develop a system for tracking expenses and bookkeeping.

▶ Set up a service for credit card processing.

Liability

▶ Draft a waiver and disclaimer and have a lawyer vet them.

▶ Buy or renew insurance.

▶ Consider incorporation.

Although working through the back end of your business can seem tedious or even overwhelming, it's a great problem to have: It means you are earning money as a yoga teacher! To continue coping with your success, you'll want to look at the front end of your business, too: the classes you are teaching and how you might arrange them into the most sustainable schedule, so you can serve your students for years to come.

6

Managing It All

· ·

WHEN YOU FIRST FINISH teacher training, you'll probably say an enthusiastic *yes* to every teaching offer you receive. This is good—the fastest route to being a good teacher is to teach often, in a wide variety of circumstances (studio, gym, community centers, outside, remotely), to a wide range of students with a wide range of ages, abilities, interests, and yoga experience. While it can feel like a trial by fire, adapting on the fly teaches you very quickly how to serve the people who are in front of you.

Soon, though, you'll need to take control of your teaching schedule to make it sustainable for the long haul. While you might be capable of teaching fifteen classes in one week one time, you probably don't want to be doing that week in and week out. The key to sustainability is knowing how much you can handle over time, then making strategic choices about which classes and activities are best worth your time. This can be because they feed your soul—at least one of your weekly classes should do just that—but for the most part your classes should be the most lucrative you can find, and the time you spend producing content should earn money for you. Look at the bottom line.

In order to do this, you'll need to figure a dollar amount for your time. This isn't just the pay rate you get per class; it should account for your planning and travel time as well as the time and equipment you use to produce video or other content, and it should also take into account the perks, like unlimited classes or free gym memberships, that you are receiving in any given job. It helps to write this out. You can use the following table, or create one of your own.

Envision Your Dream Schedule

To envision your dream schedule, start with a clear-eyed look at your current schedule. Create a table for each regular class you offer, which will help you figure your own hourly rate. (You'll find a template at yogateacherhandbook.com.) Also note any perks or intangibles like prestige or friendship and how recently you got a pay increase.

Job:
When:
Where:

Prep time	Travel time	Pay rate or average per class	Hourly rate (pay divided by time spent)	Perks/ intangibles/other considerations

Take an honest look at what you're getting, and note your reaction. Is it more than you realized? Less? Does it align with the intention and goals for your teaching that you laid out in chapter 3?

Compare this with what you know about your ideal schedule. Are you an early bird or a night owl? Do you do better powering through two or three back-to-back classes or giving yourself rest after every class? Your reaction will direct you toward things you might need to change.

Sometimes, looking at your in-person schedule with clear eyes will prompt you to generate online content, freeing you from the need to be in any particular place at any particular time. If you would like to move into this realm, add to your dream schedule: time for setup, recording, editing, and promoting your online classes, along with a projection of what you expect to earn from this work. If you are already doing such work, take a good look at how much time you're spending on it and what you're earning per hour.

You can then start to design, and maybe even to map out on a calendar, what your ideal schedule would look like. As you mold your schedule to fit your personal needs, seek to arrange it in stacks and prongs.

STACKS

A *stack* occurs on a day when you wear your yoga clothes for more than one thing. This might be teaching two classes back-to-back or, less optimally, one in the morning and one in the evening. Or it might be teaching one and taking one immediately afterward, or vice versa. The former is ideal, since you can turn off your teaching brain when you are a student; in the latter scenario, you may find yourself planning your upcoming class. If you must teach immediately after taking a class, consider sitting for meditation instead of doing savasana at the end of the class you take. You can also plan to record content before or after teaching in person.

Stacks help preserve your energy: They maximize your return on travel time and fuel, and they minimize your laundry load! This increased efficiency will let you have a day or more when you *aren't* involved in studio yoga. Having some true downtime on off days will help you refill your well of enthusiasm for your on days.

PRONGS

If you are teaching classes to a similar population—for example, a flow class on weekday mornings—work to schedule them on nonconsecutive days. That makes a *prong*. While you may not have the same students on back-to-back days, offering a Tuesday/Thursday class or a Monday/Wednesday class or any other nonconsecutive combination can draw the same students to your class more frequently.

This works especially well when you have more than one class at the same location, but it can also apply if you teach at a studio and at a gym. While students who take yoga as part of their gym membership don't usually venture beyond the gym, your more loyal students might take classes with you both at the gym and at the studio, especially if the studio class suits their schedule.

If you teach in prongs and have many regular students, you don't need to devise a completely different class every time. Students value repetition. If someone comes to your Thursday class after doing your planned sequence with you on Tuesday, don't apologize! Spin it like this: "Great to see you again! You'll see a similar sequence to Tuesday, and its familiarity will let you feel it better in your body. But pay attention: A few things will be different!"

When I taught the same sequence in multiple classes, I often had students come expressly because they wanted to repeat the class. In fact, this happened so often that I would wrap up classes by saying, "If this sequence felt especially useful to you, or if you'd like to have another crack at it, join me later this week . . ."

DAYS OFF

You serve your students best when you are feeling rested and excited to teach. If you phone it in, your energy will dull your class and negatively affect your students' experience. To feel fresh, you *must* schedule downtime and days off. This is especially important if you work a day job and teach before or after work and on weekends.

Working on the standard of the two-day weekend, I suggest you have two days per week when you do not have to wear yoga clothes, head to the studio, or practice in public. (If you enjoy a hearty physical yoga practice, at least one of these should be a fully asana-free day, to give your body time to recover.) Initially, you may not be able to have these as back-to-back days, or as Saturday and Sunday; that's OK. Work toward having them in a two-day block, even if that is Tuesday and Wednesday. Having two days off in a row is the best way to let your body and mind regenerate.

If you share your home with a partner and/or children, let at least one of these days be the same as your partner's or kids' days off. Maybe you don't want to have it be both! A day to yourself, with time to pursue exactly what feeds your soul, is the very best way to recharge so you can help people better.

Schedule Your Rest

Just as you need to envision your ideal work schedule, you should envision your ideal rest schedule. Calendar your downtime like you do your work! What would your best rest protocol look like? Is it days off? Massage? Time with friends? A weekly movie matinee? Write it down, then put it on the calendar.

TEND YOUR GARDEN

As the Yoga Sutra tells us, practice becomes firmly rooted when it is attended to for a long time without breaks. The same thing goes for your class. It takes three months to know if a class is DOA, and more than nine, sometimes a full year, to know if it's going to be viable. The best thing you can do to help your class grow roots is to be there tending it every single week. Try not to have a sub for over 10 percent of your classes. If you have travel plans or conflicts that mean you can't be there for every class for nine months, maybe a short-term series or a one-off workshop is better, or focus on online content and stick to subbing instead. Also, if you have a job that keeps you late or children who might get sick overnight, try to accept class slots at times when you know you have a backup helper at work or at home, so you can get to the studio even when contingencies happen.

Show up to teach unless you may be contagious. Cramps? Light sniffles from allergies? Ankle sprain? Show up and teach anyway. If you can't demo, bring an assistant or ask a student to set up front and center as a visual reference. (I've done this in the day or two after running ultramarathons, when I had the energy to teach but my ability to get up and down off the floor with any grace was gone.)

As a studio owner, I have heard some really awful reasons for subs. Two memorable ones: "I'm going on a trip tomorrow and haven't packed yet, so I need a sub for tonight" and "The moon just isn't right for me." When you need to ask for a sub, say only what is necessary in your appeal and no more. "I have food poisoning"—sure. But there's no need to detail your symptoms.

When you are given a new class, it's smart to get to know the teachers who offer the classes immediately before and after yours—they may be able to help out in the case of a true emergency. Be sure you store their contact information in your phone. Beyond them, identify who among the studio staff would be the best fit to sub your class, and develop a relationship with them. Invite them to your class, go to theirs, and turn to them first when you have a (rare, ideally) scheduled vacation.

SUBSTITUTES

When you do need a sub, it's smart to choose one from among your regular students—get a colleague to come to your class. Then students have continuity, and they will know this teacher from previous classes. If you like, you can even have your sub do a guest slot teaching a part of your class, so students learn to love the sub's teaching and look forward to taking class while you are away.

This is a good way to put a positive spin on having a substitute teacher. It also shows that you are planning your absence carefully, instead of indiscriminately subbing out your class. I think it's smart to tell your students when you'll have a sub, but if you find this means the attendance plummets when you are away—especially if your sub is paid per head—you may prefer not to mention it.

Depending on the studio culture, you may pay your sub out of pocket, they may be paid at your going rate, or they may receive a different rate. Be clear on what you are asking of a sub before approaching them to cover your class.

When you substitute for a colleague, give a quick introduction of yourself and mention your regular classes, so students know where they can find you. Without apologizing for being you—that is, for not being Bryan!—contextualize why you do things the way you do. With an explanation like that, your students will appreciate the opportunity to experience a new spin on the class. Ideally, you'll have been to the class before, so you should be aware of student expectations. When you bid your students goodbye, remind them where they can find you if they want to seek out your class.

Cancellations

Sometimes there's a real emergency and you cannot be present, nor can you find a sub—or, if you are teaching online, there are insurmountable technical problems. When this happens, take any steps you can to alert your students that class is canceled. It would be polite to give anyone who shows up a complimentary class in the future. If you are hosting your own classes, you'll have full say about this; if you're teaching elsewhere, the studio or venue will decide. Do your very, very best never to cancel, as it irreparably damages student confidence in you in unquantifiable ways. That said, when you're stranded by the side of the road or in the emergency room, or a storm has knocked out your power just before a live online class, your students will understand.

HANDLING SMALL CLASSES

Be clear on what constitutes a class. Some places, including my studios, say that one student can constitute a class. We do, however, offer the solo student a choice, phrased like this: "Our policy is that one person makes a class, but I realize you may not be in the mood for a private lesson. Would you like to continue, or save your class credit for next time?" If the student chooses the former, depending on your experience with them and your comfort in deviating from the class plan you've prepared, you may be able to tailor a practice to suit your student's needs. I once taught a single-person class to a student who'd come to the studio immediately after dropping off her mother at assisted living. She really needed and appreciated her yoga practice that day. Often these unintended private lessons are the most gratifying to teach.

On the other hand, if the student declines, don't take it personally. People come to group exercise classes to be with a group! The dynamic can be weird if the student isn't expecting a private lesson. Give them room to pass.

Class attendance is predictable only in part, and it fluctuates with the day of the week, the seasons, and the greater picture of what is happening locally, nationally, and even globally. We find that beautiful weather, especially the first pretty day after a stretch of hot or cold temperatures, correlates with a drop in class numbers. Don't be disheartened if you have a week or two of unusually low numbers. If you're in a university town, as I am, you'll see numbers change with the semester—midterms, breaks—and with the football or basketball team schedules.

If low numbers are a trend and you continually find yourself with class sizes of one or two, talk to your management about ways to incentivize new students. These could include offering a special deal (like a month of classes for the price of three, or two) or inviting a few friends to come to class for free to seed the room. My business partner and I cite the term "empty-restaurant syndrome." People want to be where other people are, and while a restaurant may have the very best cuisine in town, and a class might be absolutely wonderful, it's odd for patrons when they are the only ones there. Having other customers makes the restaurant or the class seem more desirable.

Check also that what you are teaching matches the description students read online, and ask a trusted friend for feedback on your teaching in the underattended class.

HANDLING LARGE CLASSES

At the other end of the spectrum, you may find yourself with classes that are near or at capacity for the room. This is a nice problem to have! If your class is regularly big and it's been near capacity for a month or more, you may need to take one or more of the following approaches.

Require Preregistration

You may need to require students to preregister. When you impose this rule, make it clear whether you will allow them to "early cancel," which means that their class credit reverts to their account, or whether all cancellations are "late cancels," which means no refunds. Studios can set their own policies about what constitutes an early cancel: It could be up to twenty-four, twelve, or two hours before the class, after which a cancellation is deemed a late cancel.

Either way, you might take a waitlist. Scheduling software can make this easy: It adds students as slots open up and alerts them to their addition. Another approach is to skip the waitlist and allow a handful of students to show up in the hopes of getting in on a standby basis. Your host may have a standard procedure. If you're the one making the policy, you'll need to experiment to see what best suits your student base.

Add a Class

Sometimes a big class can be split into two classes, perhaps back-to-back (which lets you do one class preparation for both). If you're paid per class, this is a way to serve the students while improving your bottom line. If you are being paid per head, recognize that you might divide your numbers across two classes instead of keeping them condensed in one class. Trial and error will help you get it right.

Add an Assistant

If your room fills up but you're still trying to squeeze in a few more students, having an assistant can help a lot. Between you and this helper, you can shepherd students into a tighter mat arrangement, increasing capacity. Then the assistant can float through the room, delivering props, offering demos, and, when appropriate, giving verbal and manual assists. It can be very helpful to have a second set of eyes on the students in a full room, and between the two of you, you have a better chance of offering individual attention so the students have the same personalized experience they would in a smaller class.

Add a Live Stream

If your studio offers video classes or is willing to try, you could add a live stream of the class, so students can follow along from home. When live streaming a large class, it's useful to have an assistant handle the camera duties, so you can give the students your full attention. Set up your camera toward the front of the room, with one to three students in focus, so there will always be a demonstration, even if you are moving through the room off-camera. (We will cover video in chapter 7.) These students should sign a model release form. If it's tough to get students who *want* to be on camera, offering a free class sometimes does the trick—and you may include your assistant. Be sure the studio charges for the class, and if you are new to streaming, discuss how you will be paid.

Ask for More Money

If you are hosting a class yourself, once it's been full for a month or more, raise the rates by a few dollars. You might announce that this will happen in a few weeks so that your current students have a chance to buy a package at the current rates.

If you're teaching in a gym or studio, point out your consistently full class to your manager and ask whether it might be time for a raise.

ASKING FOR A RAISE

When you are feeling busy or your classes are full, it may be time to ask for a pay raise, especially if it has been a year or two since your last increase, or if you have recently upgraded your credentials by completing a specialty training keyed to what you teach or have become an E-RYT 200, RYT 500, or E-RYT 500. All of these are entry points to a discussion with your manager or studio owner about your hourly rate. So are specific contributions you've made to the studio, like bringing in a new population of students or subbing liberally and cheerfully. Likewise, any contributions to the field, like publishing a book, developing a new volunteer program to bring yoga to underserved populations, or the like are worth mentioning in your discussion of your pay rate.

Before you ask for a raise, do your research. What is the going rate in the area? Have you hit the benchmarks set for you when you were hired or at your last pay raise, if they were explicit? Does the studio seem to be on solid financial footing? Sometimes management puts up a good front but the money is just not there.

I suggest raising the issue in an email that offers a phone call or in-person meeting with your manager. This introduces the topic while letting your manager consider whether there is room in the budget to pay you more. Your message could look like this.

> *Dear* [*Manager*],
>
> *What a continual pleasure it is to be teaching at Carolina Yoga Company! In the three years that I've been on the schedule, I've taught over 600 hours at the studio and upgraded my Yoga Alliance registry to E-RYT 200. As you know, I'm enrolled in the studio's 500-hour teacher training, and I've served as the assistant for two of Sage's intensives, helping with setup and support.*
>
> *To help fund this education, I'd like to discuss raising my per-head rate to $5.50/hour from its current $4.50 [or my per-class rate from $30 to $35—whatever feels right].*
>
> *Would you like to meet to discuss this possibility and my contributions to the studio? I'd love to get together for coffee or, if it's simpler, schedule a phone call or drop in early for your class.*

There are other ways to increase your average pay per class to free up energy, if not generate more money. Depending on the pay structure at the place or places where you work, you may be able to combine two classes into one without losing many students. If you're being paid per head, this is one way to increase your payment per hour. This extra money frees up time for you to give yoga away to needy populations and to continue your own personal studentship and practice. It makes you the best, most professional yoga teacher you can be.

There are also things your studio might do for you beyond increasing your pay. For example, your manager might offer you a free continuing education workshop or arrange a scholarship trade for you to take a training at another studio in exchange for sending one of their teachers to a workshop at your studio. Or you could receive some extra support in class: an assistant to help manage your mats, an extra desk worker to handle check-in and to cover all your nonteaching chores.

HANDLING BURNOUT

Nothing is more normal than feeling uninspired—or even unmotivated—to teach. In fact, I feel this way before almost every class, and I have come to recognize it as an expression of my nerves. I want to serve my students well, I am lightly anxious about doing a good job, and for me this translates into not feeling like teaching. But the moment class begins, this feeling goes away for me! On the day it doesn't, I will need to give myself a sabbatical: to step away from teaching, if only for a week or two of vacation, and find ways to get my mojo back.

When you feel burned out on yoga, your immediate reaction should be to go into urgent self-care mode. Carve out time for more sleep. Eat well. Hydrate. Dial back your obligations and scale back the hours you spend practicing rigorous asana or undertaking other exercise. Choose gentle and restorative yoga over challenging practices. Turn to things that regularly inspire you, whether that is spending time with friends, time in nature, or time reading.

As part of this preemptive self-care, get back to the basics of why you love yoga. Revisit a class with your original teacher. Try a mellow class at a new studio, or something fresh online. Reread the writing you were prompted to do in part 1 of this book. Talk to your mentors about how you're feeling. If the mood persists, talk to a professional therapist. You don't need to be up all the time. Inspiration waxes and wanes.

HANDLING COMPETITION

Even with the explosion of yoga over the last decades and the expansion of video content online, there are still many more people not practicing yoga than who currently are. There is certainly enough of a student base for every yoga teacher to find a group of people to help. This may not always be in a studio, which by definition has a more limited group of potential students coming through. It might instead mean you seek out places where you can share your teachings outside of conventional methods: schools, community centers, prisons. Remember that there is abundance waiting for you if your goal is simply to share yoga.

If your goal is to earn money teaching yoga, you'll sometimes bump up against competition. This could be vying with another teacher or many other teachers for a prime-time slot, an invitation to a festival, or even social media followers or sponsorships. Or it could be noticing another teacher who seems to be crushing it in your online niche. Comparison is the thief of joy! When you find yourself feeling envious of another teacher, you have a special opportunity to undergo some self-study about the root of your feelings. This can prompt you to next steps to develop your own skill set to move closer to what you want for yourself.

Sometimes you perceive competition because a teacher or a studio seems to be following a little too closely in your footsteps—for example, offering workshops on topics similar to yours, maybe even using language that's very like what you use. Or maybe it's using imagery or music or sequencing similar to what you are offering. Often, this truly has nothing to do with you. Or it could be a flattering imitation: Someone sees your success and tries to emulate it. If it seems to be a more deliberate poaching of your creative content, take a careful look while giving the perceived competition the benefit of the doubt. Is it feasible this isn't about you? If you still believe it is, talk to your yoga mentors before approaching your colleague to discuss the issue.

Often the best response is to focus more clearly on yourself and your own goals. When you are faced with a sense of competition, revisit the writing you did in part 1 of this book. Get in touch with who you are as a teacher, who your students are, and how you can help them in your own unique way. If you can stay in your own lane and focus on being the best version of your authentic self that you can be, your students will find you, and they will appreciate you for exactly who you are and what you have to share.

LEAVING A REGULAR JOB

What happens when you are ready to move on? If the studio has a regular schedule-change window, alert the owner and/or manager shortly before the window opens, so they have a chance to begin thinking about who will be the best replacement for you. Based on your subs and students, you may have suggestions for a replacement, but do not speak to your potential replacement until you have talked to your manager. The management may want to take the class in a different direction. This is their prerogative and should be their choice, not yours.

If you have online content housed at the studio site, refer to your contract about whether it will continue to be available—and whether you will be paid for it, and how. The circumstances of your departure will likely affect the outcome: If you are taking a maternity leave and plan to return, it will likely stay online; if you are terminated or leaving to open your own studio or to teach for the competition, it will likely not.

Make sure you are clear on the terms of your noncompetition clause, if you signed one. These may cover a limited range and a limited period of time. Even if you did not agree to such a clause in your contract, be sensitive and canny about where you agree to teach after leaving your current position. You may wind up hurting feelings and closing a door to future employment. Use your best judgment and your mentor's advice when making such choices. You'll want to decide how much to share with your current employer about why you're leaving. If it's corporate culture, is that something they might change with carefully expressed feedback? If it's just money, be prepared for your current host to offer you a raise, and consider whether you'd stay in that case. You'll want to be careful about committing to a new place before seeing whether your current employer might match your offer.

Depending on the situation and the studio culture, you may be asked to leave immediately when you give your notice, so be prepared for this outcome. It is often not a personal choice from the business side, but simply because when things are changing it can be smoothest to change them immediately.

Talk to your employer about when and whether you or they will let your students know that you have moved on and to where. This varies case by case, and it's best to ask and to be sure you understand the answer. Do *not* use the studio software to access students' contact information—that is a breach of the students' privacy and some managers may see it as theft, since the information belongs to the business, not the teacher. If you are leaving for another studio, especially if you are teaching a similar class at the same time, do not expect that your soon-to-be-ex-employer will let you announce this in class. If you are taking a sabbatical or an indefinite maternity leave, you may be welcome to mention this in class.

Depending on the circumstances of your departure, you may not be able to let your students know. Naturally, you would want them to find you in your new location even if you can't expressly mention it, which is why it's good to have an online presence that makes your schedule easy to find. You can post your new schedule on your social media and, of course, on your website, as well as on your newsletter list. Following the promotional advice from chapter 4 will make you easy for students to find.

Now that you've thought through the teacher you want to be, how you'll express that to employers and students, what you want your workweek to look like, and how your business will be structured, it's time to think through what you do in your interactions with students in your regular weekly classes.

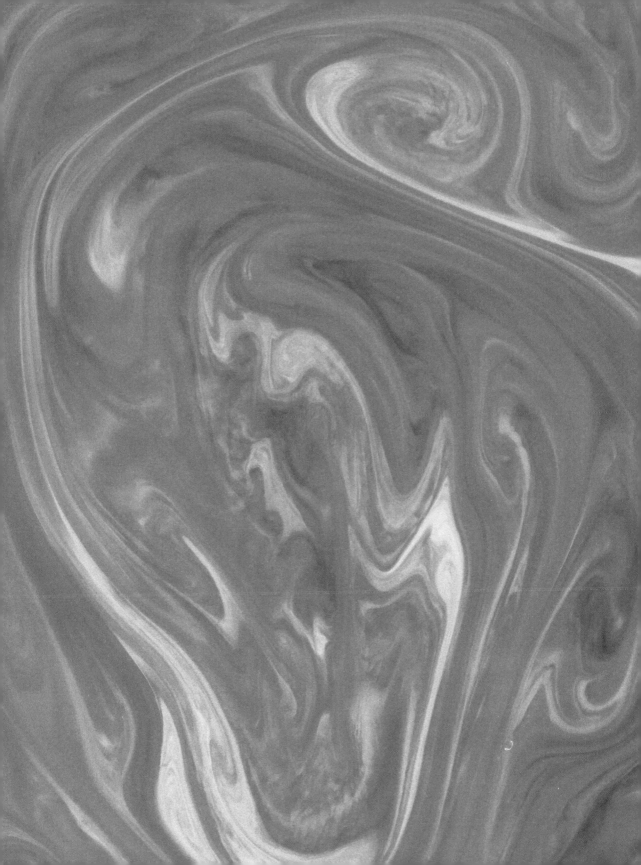

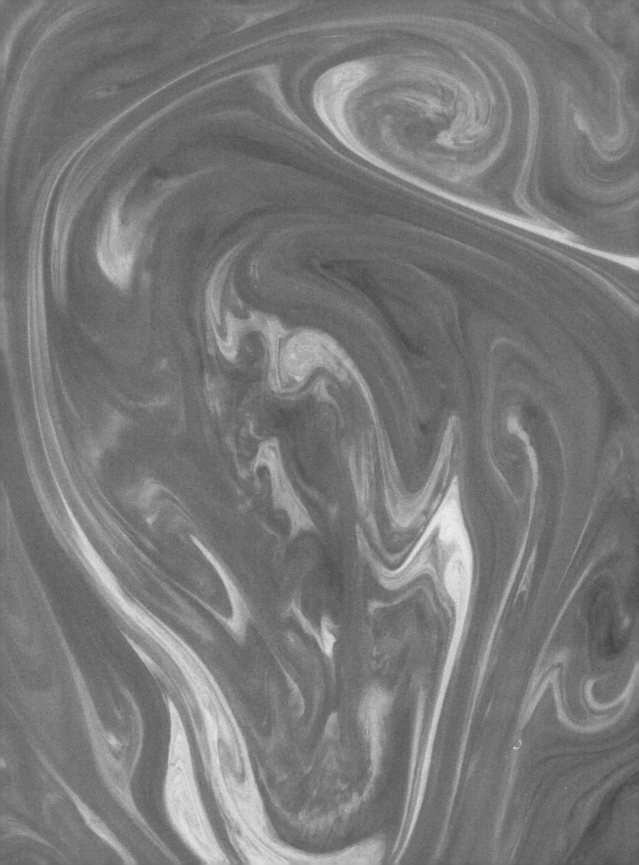

PART 3

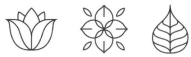

Hosting a Class

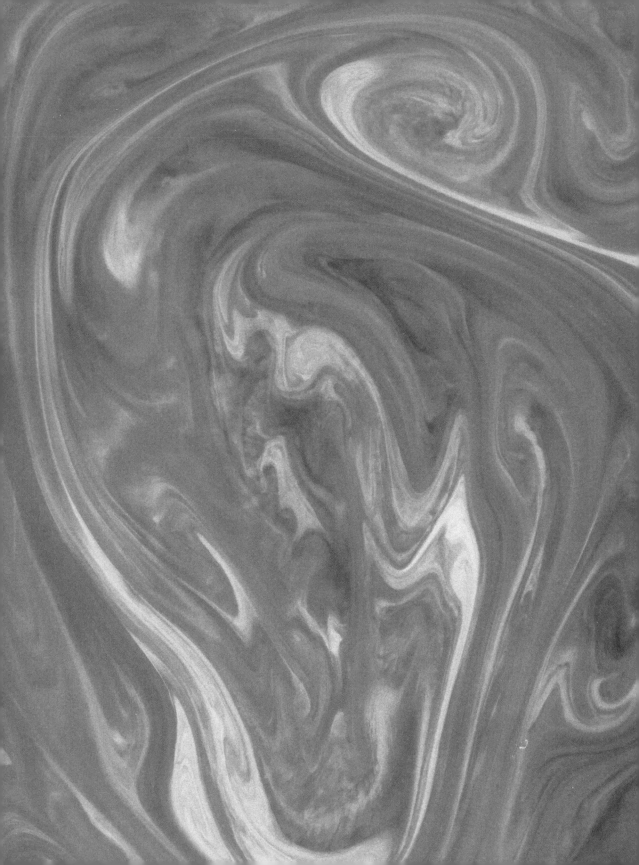

7

Developing Your Class: Planning and Reflection

· ·

WHETHER YOU'RE A NEW TEACHER getting your feet under you or an experienced one looking to get to the next level, focusing on the fundamentals—what happens in the standard daily yoga class—will make you the best teacher you can be. Just as regular revisiting of your reasons for teaching yoga and your vision for your career will keep you on track, so will regular attention to the tone you are setting in every class and diligent reflection and self-evaluation to ensure you are being the teacher you want to be.

Our project here is to explore how you can make the best use out of the time you have outside the classroom, to perfect and refine your time spent in the classroom. I'll take you through how best to plan for your class, and give you tips on how best to reflect on your teaching, so that each class is better than the last. We will also cover how to set up for recording live and staged classes.

We'll start with how you can be a gracious host for your guests—your students—and consider how to set the scene to create the right mood to guide your class into satisfying inner awareness. Along the way, it's helpful to think of teaching a yoga class as hosting a dinner party.

CHOOSE THE GUESTS

It's not a party without guests! If you're subbing or taking over an existing class, learn who the typical students are. What is their yoga experience? How old are they? Why do they come to yoga? Knowing who the regulars are and where their tastes lie will dictate how you plan your class. When you can, take the class in the weeks before you begin teaching it. Carefully read the class description and begin to think about how you will meet your students' expectations.

Whether you are creating a new class, adding a new class to the schedule, or creating your own teaching opportunities, put special thought into who your ideal students are. What is their age, level of experience, desire for yoga? Will they want a playful teacher or a serious one? What do they have in common? What is a problem they might have, like high stress, tight hamstrings, or back pain, that yoga can solve? Answering these questions will not only help you prepare the class; it will help you with scheduling and marketing, as we have seen. It may be useful to jot down some notes. Take these notes to your hiring manager and ask if you are on the right track. The better your class can serve your students from day one, the happier and more loyal they will be.

Describe Your Students

Whether you're taking over an existing class or starting a new one, take some time to think about the students you may meet on the mat. Ask yourself, your hiring manager, or the teacher you're taking over from:

▶ How old is the typical student?

▶ How much experience does the typical student have?

▶ Why does this student come to yoga?

▶ How can yoga help this student? (This will help you plan your sequence.)

Satisfaction = Perception – Expectations

One of our teachers also teaches business classes at the University of North Carolina Kenan-Flagler Business School. There, she told me, she tells her students that customer satisfaction follows this formula: Satisfaction = Perception – Expectations. Satisfaction is a result of what the consumer perceived they received minus what they expected to receive. Satisfaction is positive when your students' experience is equal to or better than what they thought they would get, and negative when their expectations exceed their reality.

One way to manage expectations is by writing a very clear class description that lets students know what they will experience in the class. At Carolina Yoga Company, each class description also includes ratings of challenge and chill on a scale from 0 to 5. Restorative Yoga then gets a challenge level of 0 and a chill level of 5, while Flow Yoga has a challenge of 3 or 4 and a chill of 2. Flow and Unwind has a challenge of 3 or 4 but a chill of 4, because it ends in a restorative pose. Adding such a scale might help you manage students' expectations.

PLAN THE MENU

The first step in class planning is to unroll your mat with a notebook or laptop handy. Take a moment to get centered, and remember your intention as a yoga teacher. Take another moment to visualize your students and recognize what they need from the practice. These needs and your intention will guide you as you create your class.

Decide where the home base for your warm-up will be: reclining, prone, seated, hands and knees, or standing. Slot in moves to take the spine in every direction: forward and back, left and right, round and round. Find ways to expand and contract this sequence to make it longer and shorter, and note modifications for different bodies and injuries. Write it all down.

For example, here is a classic warm-up sequence that starts from hands and knees:

▶ Cat/cow
▶ Child's pose with side stretch
▶ Thread-the-needle twist

Your notes might eventually look like:

- ▶ Cat/cow
  - ▪ Wrist issues: forearms to blocks
  - ▪ Knee pressure: blanket under knees
  - ▪ Full alternative: standing cat/cow
- ▶ Child's pose with side stretch
  - ▪ Knee issues: blanket between calves and thighs
  - ▪ Knees closer or wider to suit each body
  - ▪ Option to support forehead on a block
- ▶ Thread-the-needle twist
  - ▪ Sweeter: palm or elbow to floor, kick L leg to side when twisting to L
  - ▪ Spicier: drop to shoulder, raise arm, half-bind arm, raise leg
- ▶ Variations
  - ▪ Return to cat/cow between subsequent poses, add a plank or down dog, repeat each move two to five times (can grow from a three-minute sequence to a ten-minute sequence this way)
  - ▪ Try the side stretch and twist from child's pose, hands and knees, and belly-down positions; let students choose
  - ▪ Interesting to return to these moves later in class, too

Then move on and do the same for standing poses, mat poses, and finishing poses. If you're not sure what to put in here, you might find inspiration in my book *Everyday Yoga*.

Next find transitions between each of the sequences you've planned. How will students come off the floor for your standing segment of class? How will they get back down to the floor? What are some options to work around common injuries? Write all these down.

At this point, you'll have a lot of notes. Taking something this long into class would lead you to refer to your notes too often while you teach. Now find a way to condense this—perhaps titles for the sequences will work better, or stick-figure drawings, or whatever shorthand makes sense to you.

Recognize What Comes Easy

If you've never eaten a restrictive diet because of allergies, sensitivities, or ethical choice, you've never had to think about ways to plan a meal to avoid all the potential hazards and pitfalls—lucky you! Similarly, your greatest strengths as a student can translate into your biggest weaknesses as a teacher. The things that come naturally to you can prove very hard to teach, as you haven't had to go through the steps of learning them. If you're flexible, you can have problems understanding how frustrating it is for those who aren't. If you're strong, you won't remember the modifications that help students develop their own strength.

If you find that ease in asana comes quite naturally to you, try doing something else that does challenge you: Take a CrossFit class, sign up for cooking lessons, learn a new sport. This will remind you that some learning curves are steep, and it will keep you compassionate.

This blind spot applies to all your physical gifts from birth—not just flexibility, or strength, but having a thin body, or smaller breasts, or female rather than male genitalia. An ample belly, bigger boobs, or a penis and testicles can make some poses tough to find comfort in. (Many men don't love eagle pose or cow-face pose!) Cast a caring, sympathetic eye around the room, both when you teach and when you are a student in class, and imagine ways you can modify poses for every body type. Then talk to your students—if not your walk-in students, your friends, your partner, or your private clients—about their comfort in a variety of poses. Better yet, read a book or take a training on how to adapt yoga to different bodies. Jessamyn Stanley's *Every Body Yoga* and Kimberly Carson and Carol Krucoff's *Relax into Yoga for Seniors* are two great resources.

Beyond the physical privilege you have, recognize the other privileges you bear: These could be privileges of socioeconomic status, gender identity, sexual orientation, or race. You are very lucky to be someone with the free time and the resources to pursue yoga practice and yoga teacher training; many are not. Be open to ways you can make yoga a more inclusive practice for people from every background. Many yoga studios draw a rich, white, thin clientele, and you may land in one of these. Great: You can use the income you earn there to free you up to offer classes in community centers, schools, churches, rape or youth crisis shelters, or wherever your heart draws you. This is the yogic principle of *seva*, selfless service. To maximize your impact, focus on bringing yoga *to* the underserved communities—meeting people where they are, at the point of their need—rather than offering free classes at a studio, which will likely never come to the attention of the students you're targeting.

Develop Plan B

No matter how much careful thought you give to who your students are, one or more will often challenge your ability to adapt on the fly. Think of this as having a dinner guest with a food allergy or an aversion: It's good to have something in the pantry in case your planned menu doesn't work.

Once I invited a successful restaurateur and her husband for dinner. Only when they arrived did she mention he was vegetarian! Happily, it was an easy fix not to garnish the gnocchi with prosciutto. While you can't please all of the people all of the time, especially when you are a new teacher, be sure to keep some back-pocket poses and sequences that will work for virtually anybody. Say you have people in class with wrist, shoulder, knee, and toe injuries. Instead of lots of hands and knees on the floor, for example, you could lead a class that has standing poses but little time coming up from and down to the floor.

Theme It—or Not

Consider whether you would like to add a theme to your class. If so, write it out and consider collecting some quotes, chants, or songs to support your theme. You'll find a full explanation of weaving a theme into class in my book *Teaching Yoga Beyond the Poses*, cowritten with Alexandra DeSiato. If you naturally and spontaneously find theming easy, please forge ahead! If you don't, choose one simple lesson for all your classes as you get started teaching. This could be mindful awareness in the present moment or finding the right balance between effort and ease. Each of these is a lovely theme. Bring the theme into all your classes, and your students will benefit. Over time, you'll grow more comfortable weaving a wide range of inspiration into your classes. Talking about points from yoga philosophy is one approach. One of my favorites is unpacking the concept of *samskara* as either a groove or a rut. Another easy one is keying to the seasons—you can structure a class for autumn around surrender, with ample tree poses and a lesson about letting go of what you don't need now. Theming is a lovely way to take students deeper. If you're a new teacher, you may want to wait to experiment with theming until you have more experience. (The same thing goes for assists; we teach them as part of our advanced studies yoga teacher training, instead of our 200-hour YTT.)

Time It

Now practice your sequence to be sure it's appropriate for the amount of time allotted for your class. This is a good time to reread the class description and be sure the menu you've planned jibes with it. Just as you wouldn't try out a new dish on guests you're trying to impress—your partner's boss, say—you shouldn't arrive at class unsure about how to cue your sequence or take the poses in it. Practice, practice, practice. Depending on what works best for your nerves and your delivery style, you might practice the entire class in real time, speaking everything aloud, from your intro to your cues, as you move through the sequence or guide a friend or colleague through the practice. Or you might try your sequence as your home practice, without describing what you're doing out loud. As you go, think of ways you can expand or contract the sequence if the timing proves to be different once you're teaching it to live students.

Think of this practice as doing your *mise en place*, a French kitchen term that refers to putting things into place. In a commercial kitchen, each cook sets up their station with the tools, food, and condiments they will need for the shift. This varies from station to station and from kitchen to kitchen, but the process is common to every successful enterprise.

Collate Your Class Plans

Design several classes using whatever format best suits your planning style. Consider:

▶ Who are your students?

▶ What do they need to learn?

▶ Is there a theme to weave in to the class?

▶ Where will the class start: seated, reclining, standing?

▶ What are your planned sequences?

▶ How will you modify these for injury?

Look at the big picture: Is the planned sequence a balanced diet? Do students move forward and back, left and right, round and round? Does the plan skew too much toward standing, or sitting, or reclining? Tweak your plans until they feel organically balanced.

While it may make sense for the first draft of these plans to be written on paper, I suggest finding a software program that works for you—ideally one that's stored in the cloud. You may be more of a spreadsheet thinker or more of a free-form notes or sketches thinker: Whatever makes sense is great. But having your class plans available in the cloud means you'll never be without them, and you'll be able to mix and match easily over time. If you write in a notebook, snap a photo of your plans or scan them, and save those images in the cloud. If you lose your notebook, you won't lose all your work.

Exactly what your plans look like will depend on what works best for you. You might write the name of each pose, including a few key cues. You might draw your sequence using stick figures. You might simply jot down a few phrases that, in your mind, unspool into full segments of class. Only you know the best way to do this. Be creative and intuitive, and you'll be fine.

Teaching Poses You Can't Do

Would you serve your guests something you hadn't tasted? Probably not, if you want them to have the best experience possible. Before important dinner parties, you might even do a test run or two, so you can smooth out any bumps and feel really confident in your execution of the recipe. Similarly, you shouldn't lead your students into poses, especially deep stretching or balancing poses, that you haven't gained your own confidence with yet.

There are exceptions here. I have an aversion to olives, but I don't hesitate to set out olives as an appetizer. When I do, they go alongside other snack options, like nuts. People can choose them or not. If you are teaching a group of experienced practitioners, it's OK to give them free rein to express the poses as they like within the context of the group experience. By that I mean they might add an arm bind or some other flourish, while still generally following the outline of the sequence as you are cuing it.

Perhaps a pose was once a regular part of your repertoire but because of an injury you aren't practicing it these days. (For example, after a total knee replacement, you may never sit in a kneeling position or hero pose again.) It would be fine to lead that pose, with a word or two about why you will not be demonstrating it.

SET THE TABLE

Once you have your menu planned and your ingredients prepared, it's time to think about the space where your meal will be served. The choices you make before students arrive to class are some of the most important in setting the tone for their experience. It's analogous to a hostess choosing decorations and music, creating the ambience with lighting and scents, and preparing the physical space for the dinner party.

If you are teaching online, you may have total control over your set. Depending on where you're teaching in person, you may or may not be able to control some or all of the contingencies of the classroom. But thinking through the mood you'd like to set beforehand will help you reduce your nerves and create the most welcoming atmosphere for your class.

If You Are Using a Camera

If you are video-recording a class with students in it, think through exactly what this will involve, as far in advance as you can. Consider adding "(Camera)" to the class title and a line to the class description that explains how much of the room is on camera and whether the class is streamed live or available for viewing on demand. This will help manage students' expectations of the experience.

Most importantly, test and double-test your equipment, which will depend on your camera setup. You'll want to set your camera on a tripod. Determine where that tripod can go to capture you and, if appropriate, a few students for demonstrations without having a detrimental effect on the experience of the students in the room who do not want to be on camera.

You'll almost always want to record in landscape mode (horizontal) rather than portrait (vertical)—Instagram video is one possible exception. Shooting in landscape mode allows you to frame your shots best, if you are demonstrating asana.

For live streaming online. You will need a camera and a streaming service. A phone camera, especially for a newer, high-end phone, will offer better quality than the built-in camera on a laptop or tablet. You can stream via many different platforms, from Facebook Live to Vimeo Premium. If the decision is yours, choose one that will let you use the rear-facing camera on your phone (not the front-facing selfie camera, which has generally lower quality). If you want to use your computer to see the students who are watching live, there are various third-party apps that will let you use your phone's HD camera as a webcam. You can also stream from your phone while joining the meeting from your computer; that way, you can both generate high-quality video and pull the online students into the classroom, if only virtually. When you are live streaming, turning off all other devices on the Wi-Fi network helps ensure your signal is strong. See my service and app recommendations at yogateacherhandbook.com.

For recordings to be played on demand. Record using either your phone's rear-facing camera (with settings turned to 4K or as high as they will go) or an SLR camera with a large storage capacity. Check the amount of storage available on your phone before you begin. You may use a third-party app, such as MovieBox Pro (on Android) and ProMovie Recorder (on iOS devices), to tweak exposure and focus settings and to see how much recording space is free. Upload your files from the phone or SD card to the cloud as soon as you can.

Once you have tested and finalized where the camera will go, you can make informed decisions about all of the factors described in what follows.

Cameras Complicate Class

I've done lots of different video shoots over the last dozen years—generating hundreds of hours of DVD and streaming video content—including dedicated video shoots with and without students demonstrating, recorded classes for play-on-demand, and live-streaming classes. They are all stressful to teach, especially the last two. Recording an open class with paying students creates a suboptimal experience for everyone, because the teacher is working to serve two groups at once: the students who are there in the room *and* the ones who are watching live or will be watching later. While such classes can be a stopgap solution to help a studio's bottom line in periods of social distancing, they are very difficult on the teacher. When the teacher is overly challenged, the quality of the teaching suffers, and the students have a less-than-ideal experience.

Whenever possible, I prefer a scheduled shoot that is not a regular class— and with dedicated camera and sound techs, if you can afford that, or a friend to help with these logistics. If you need students to demonstrate, ask some teacher colleagues or your regulars and have them model in exchange for the class. You'll produce a better result, and your content will be more helpful for viewers.

Arrival

Arrive early! You can't be a centered, calm leader for your class if you are squealing in late and frazzled. Aim to arrive at least twenty minutes ahead, or more if you are in an area with frequent traffic slowdowns. Plan for problems: If you did hit unusual traffic, whom would you contact to let them know you are running late? Is their contact info readily available in your phone? What is the protocol for contacting students or, if worse comes to worst, canceling the class if you get trapped in a jam?

If parking is difficult at the studio or gym, where will you look for backup parking options? Having thought through these contingencies will allow you to be calmer should they arise.

When you arrive, take a moment to use the bathroom, wash your hands well, and take at least a few deep breaths to feel grounded. If you have the time and inclination, run through the sequence you plan, either by visualizing it or by physically moving through relevant segments. It's useful to be warmed up, especially if you are going to demonstrate for your students.

Depending on the studio policy, you may have access to a roster of students who have already signed in to the class. Review it so you can address each of them by name. Similarly, you may be able to scroll back through previous weeks to see who has been coming lately and refresh your memory of their names.

If you are teaching both in real time and on live stream, set up and check your equipment or have an assistant help with this. If you are teaching live stream from a set with no students, log in early. Check that you have fresh or well-charged batteries in your microphone!

As your students arrive, greet them warmly. Angle your body so that you can make eye contact with and smile at each student as they arrive, even if you are involved in a conversation with someone else and can't speak to them. If you are hosting a live-stream class from set, greet students as they log in. (Generally, you'll see their names, unless they are using a family member's account.) Offer a warm welcome, as you would in person. Brief students about the protocols around muting their microphones and whether to have their video displayed—these factors depend on your vision for the class as well as student comfort.

Temperature

When you have the chance to control the temperature, it's better to err on the side of being too warm than too cool. Students can generally shed a layer if they are hot. But temperatures below 70 degrees can register as too chilly for students. When their bodies perceive that it's cold, they are less likely to release into stretches. Conversely, a room that is hot can sometimes create a false sense of flexibility—be aware, and use language to keep students from pushing too hard in a warm room.

If your room is warm and your students are sweating, be attuned to the temperature as you settle in to the mat portion of class. As the teacher, you won't be generating as much heat as your students, nor will you be as still toward the end of class. If you've turned on the air-conditioning or fans during the peak of class, turn them off as you coast toward the end. In winter, consider turning the heat up so students will be warm enough in savasana.

If you can control the temperature, let it support what is happening in class. For still practices, and at the start and end of class, it's useful to have the room be warmer. But be especially aware at the end of class, because if students have sweated and their clothes are damp, they can cool off too quickly. In the active portions of class, cooler air or a fan can help keep students comfortable.

Lighting

Just as it does in a dinner party or a restaurant, lighting plays an important role in setting a mood and making your guests comfortable. While we all have personal preferences, here are some general guidelines for creating the best lighting for class.

If your studio space has natural light, such as sun shining through a window, do not set up directly in front of it or you will be backlit, which means your students will have the sun shining in their eyes. Instead, orient the room so you are well lit and the students won't have to squint to watch you demonstrate.

It's nice to teach in a space where the lights are on dimmers. You can adjust as needed to suit the time of day and mood of the section you're teaching. Turn the lights up gently at the end of class—don't slam them on all at once. If your lights are not dimmable, be aware of when the students need light to see and when the light is an annoyance pulling them out of inner experience. I've handled this issue when traveling to teach by keeping the overhead lights on for the first half of the mat sequence, then turning them off—and sometimes propping open a door for light—for the second half. If you need to do the same, when students turn to one side on the way out of savasana, ask them to cover their eyes with a forearm, then turn the lights on. That way, they'll still have their eyes closed for several moments, allowing for adjustment.

Sometimes, rooms are lit in regions—front, middle, and back—and it makes sense to keep light on your mat while darkening the students' mats. You'll have to see what works best, and don't be shy about asking your students whether they can see or would like the lights adjusted.

With some foresight, you can work around problems with lighting by bringing your own lights. This could be a string of LED fairy lights—you can get 100 yards for $30 or so online—or a spotlight (even just a desk lamp) to light your mat.

Or enhance the mood with candles. Before you use real candles, check with the management of the space where you're teaching. They may be forbidden. Either way, consider using LED-lit faux candles. They avoid any risk of fire or wax spills, are odorless and smoke-free, and cast a very sweet light.

For video classes, lighting can make the difference between something mediocre and something really great. If you are teaching meditation, breath work, or other lecture-style and talking-head classes, a small camera-mounted ring light (like you see reality stars use for selfies) will do. For full-body demonstrations, a two- or three-light rig of LED lights on stands will get you a lot of bang for your buck. Set up what videographers call the "key light" just behind the camera at the height of (or just taller than) your head, angled at your face. Natural lighting can work well as a key light, too: Set the camera with its back to the window, and position yourself facing both window and camera. Set up a second light—the fill light—in a corner, shining toward you from the side, to fill in any shadows set by the key light. If you can afford a third light, use it as a fill light from the other side. A photographer's reflector, a white wall, or even a white sheet can serve this purpose as well. Adding either barn doors to focus the light or soft boxes to diffuse it can customize the lighting to achieve different effects. Some LED lights offer both warm and cool light; be sure to match the ambient natural or electric light in the room, so color tones come out well. Visit yogateacherhandbook.com for a current list of equipment suggestions.

Smells

Some schools of yoga regularly light incense as part of the mood of the space. But students with allergies and breathing problems can find this highly irritating. Try an essential oil diffuser instead, or go without. If you must use incense, tell your students ahead of time, on your website or in your class description, so they can make an educated decision about whether to attend.

Similarly, if you are going to use essential oils on your hands during savasana or other assists, let students know in advance, and give them an easy way to opt out. People often have scent sensitivities or preferences. (I used lemongrass in my mask during a week of cadaver dissection and was immediately transported back to the lab when a teacher pressed on my shoulders with lemongrass oil on her hands!) And some oils aren't great to have on your face—think peppermint or citrus. Oil from your hands will transfer to students' clothes and hair, and while they may enjoy the smell of lavender for a moment, that doesn't mean they want to be trailing it all day.

If you really, really want to use oil for aromatherapy purposes, put the oil on your own upper arm, chest, or shoulders, and let the smell transmit during your assist. That way, students get the experience without any lingering aftereffects. The trick in this is applying the oil to your arm without getting it on your hands! A tissue can help: Apply the oil to the edge of a folded tissue, then dab it on your arm or tuck it under your collar or shoulder strap. Do *not* push the brand if it is one that you personally distribute; students do not come to class to be upsold, and many studios specifically ban such sales.

Sound

If you are recording video, setting up sound is critical. An external microphone is always superior to the default microphone on your phone or video camera. Students may watch a class with subpar lighting, framing, or video resolution—but if they can't hear you, they will click away. Depending on the room you're teaching in and your budget, your choices include:

Bluetooth earbud microphone. These are budget-friendly if you already have a pair, and they are discreet since they fit in your ear. Apple AirPods, Beats Powerbeats, and similar products will capture your voice better than your computer or phone mic. Problems will arise if the fit isn't good or your movement knocks the earbud loose, so be sure to practice before recording.

Lavalier or headset microphone with wireless transmitter and receiver. This three-piece setup involves a microphone clipped to your lapel (lavalier, sometimes shortened to "lav") or hooked around your ears (headset), with a wire that runs to a transmitter, typically clipped to the back of your waistband or worn in a belt. The transmitter then delivers the sound signal to a matching receiver, which plugs in to your camera. These are nice for recording in bigger rooms, since the mic is close to your face, reducing echoes. They can also work for amplification within the room (for example, teaching at a bigger venue with many students), if given the proper setup. One drawback to the lavalier mic is that moving your arms, which you'll often do while demonstrating, can cause your shirt fabric to brush along the microphone, causing distracting noises.

Directional ("shotgun") microphone mounted to the camera. If you are teaching in a small space or one with carpeting, and your camera will be within around 10 feet (3 m) away from you, a directional or shotgun microphone is a nice choice. It requires no hardware for you to wear, and it delivers good sound, provided you face the camera. You'll attach it to your camera or tripod with a cold shoe mount (cold means the mount is not electrified, as is a hot shoe mount for a flash attachment).

USB mic for voice over after the fact. If you aren't teaching students in person in real time, consider recording the demonstration of the practice without talking at all. This eases the burden and lets you concentrate on holding poses and sides for the appropriate length. Then, you can use video editing software to record a voiceover in a quiet room later. If your home office space isn't quiet, take a USB microphone into your closet and shut the door or build a pillow fort and cover yourself in a quilt. Both of these approximate a quiet, sound-deadened studio. They are also a good choice for recording audio-only content, like guided meditations.

Whatever microphone you are using, be sure that it is set as the chosen microphone on your camera, phone, or computer. Tap it to confirm; the audio signal display on your camera should jump. In any wireless microphone setup, radio and cell signal interference can cause pops and glitches on the audio. Record a few test sessions, and listen carefully. Wireless microphones often allow you to switch to a different frequency if there is interference. Be sure to set your cell phone (and smart watch, if you wear one) to airplane mode. If you are using your phone to transmit via Wi-Fi while you record, you can then turn the Wi-Fi back on, while keeping the cell signal off.

If you are inputting the sound from a microphone to a cell phone, you will need a few adapters to allow the transmission: One is a TRS to TRRS adapter and the second, if you are using a phone without a headphone jack, is a converter of TRRS to whatever input you do have (say, Lightning connector or Micro USB).

The last step to generating good sound is to consider people who will never hear it at all. Closed captions make your video more accessible to people with hearing impairments and those who encounter your content while scrolling online. Many video hosts like YouTube and Facebook automatically (though sometimes inaccurately) generate captions, which you can edit for precision. If you are using other platforms for your video, it's worth using YouTube Studio or a paid service like 3Play, Amara, Kapwing, or Rev to generate captions for you. Then, you can upload the captions file to your preferred video host.

Visit yogateacherhandbook.com for recommendations on equipment, editing, and captioning services at various price points.

Music

The right music can set a lovely tone for class and boost—or lower—the mood according to what you are going for. But there are several arguments against music. Here are the biggest.

Associations. Students will have an emotional reaction to music. While that can be good, it can also be bad. Consider the student who can't stand a certain genre, or who hears "their song" with a partner who just dumped them. You'll never know exactly what emotions your playlist evokes. Even if you're playing instrumental music, students can have reactions according to their own experiences. I had a playlist that included Debussy's "Clair de Lune" during savasana, and after class a student walked up and said, "Clair de Lune!" "Yes," I said, "Beautiful, right?" "Ugh! It was my piano recital piece and I get tense every time I hear it!"

Words. Lyrics can pull students away from inner experience and into the music. And you'll never realize how many expletives are in a song until you're playing it in class! If you're trying to avoid this distraction by playing Sanskrit chants, know that can be off-putting to students who don't know what the words mean.

Volume. Volume can be very difficult to get right. Depending on the sound system, students near the speaker might get a very different volume than those across the room. Personally, I find nothing more distracting than music played at a low volume. My ears prick up trying to hear it. I'm in the go-loud-or-go-home camp. But some students will have trouble hearing you if the music is too loud.

Surprises. You'll inevitably mess it up: You'll forget to put your phone on airplane mode and a call will come in; your carefully curated playlist will be on shuffle and you won't know how to turn it off; the Wi-Fi will be down or stuttering when you intended to stream your music.

Licensing. Because yoga class can be deemed a public performance, you will need to pay a royalty fee to each of the song licensing outfits, ASCAP, BMI, and SESAC, in order to be aboveboard in playing recorded songs in class. And they are relentless in their pursuit of your money! You can work around this by using royalty-free music; using a service like YogiTunes, where a subscription includes performance rights; by having live music played in class, such as classical guitar during savasana; or by skipping music entirely.

Considerations for online classes. All these arguments against using music—licensing included—apply to online classes, with some special complications. If you are teaching a class in real time, it can be hard enough to get the sound levels right on your voice. Adding music further confounds the sound mix. Often, the music comes out as just one or two random notes that viewers notice from time to time. Teachers work around this by curating and sharing playlists they suggest students play during class ("OK, everyone, if you're using the playlist, start it now!"), which also works around licensing regulations. Going without music is simpler for you, and it allows your students to enjoy the quiet or add their personal favorite soundtrack as they follow along at home.

Of course, there are many good reasons for using music in class.

Sonic buffer. If you are teaching in a gym, you may need music to create a buffer between the serene environment in the studio space and the pop hits and clanking weight plates outside. Some gyms even require you to use music, because students expect it. (If so, they should cover your licensing fees or provide you with the music.)

Set the mood. Especially at the beginning of class, as students are coming in and setting up, music can fill the space and set a relaxing tone. The dinner party analogy still holds here—if it's a good party, you only notice the music when you arrive or if there's a lull in conversation. Otherwise, it fades into the background. Consider playing some walk-in music at the start of class, and possibly a short, calming song for the first part of savasana.

Familiarize the foreign. For students who find yoga intimidating, hearing familiar popular music in class can increase their comfort level.

Ultimately, your students won't notice or care about the music as much as you do. As a former radio DJ, I used to put great effort into my playlists for studio classes. But as I traveled to teach teams on fields and in gyms, I grew used to going without music, and eventually I stopped using it entirely.

One night after class, one of my long-term regular students commented, "You didn't use music tonight."

"That's right," I replied. "And I haven't for six months."

When students are really in the zone—when they are doing yoga—their attention is focused inward, not on the music.

If you do choose to use music, consider mentioning that in the class description or keying to it in the title of your class. Some studios will display a musical note like an asterisk alongside the title of any class using music. I love this: It sets and manages students' expectations for whether there will be music in class.

Dress Code

One of my students recounted to me her scouting visit to the training facility of a National Football League team that hired her. She scoped out the room where she'd be teaching, assessed the lighting and sound, and discussed goals for her work with the players. At the end of the tour, her client said, "Let's talk dress code." "Sure," she replied, "Shorts and T-shirts are fine—what the players are wearing today will work well." "No," said the client, "I mean *your* dress code." He walked her into the equipment room, handed her a large T-shirt, and directed, "Wear this. Neutral colors: black, gray, green." Now in her fourth year of teaching the team, she reports consciously dressing modestly with "basic attire and minimal makeup."

Dressing professionally in yoga is very different from dressing professionally in virtually any other field. Skintight leggings aren't just allowed, they are the norm. So is a body-skimming top. Both make your personal practice more comfortable—no one wants a mouth full of material in downward-facing dog—and when you are teaching, they make your alignment clear to your students.

As you choose your clothing for work as a professional yoga teacher, consider the setting. What I'd wear to teach in my own studio—leggings, a tank top, and a top layer or two for warmth—might not be appropriate in other environments. In your day-to-day teaching, be aware of how much you are showing, within the parameters of typical yoga clothing and your own studio culture. While students are looking to you to see how to do a pose, they should not be distracted by extremely low-cut tops or sheer pants.

If you haven't already reached this conclusion, you'll soon realize that all yoga pants are sheer under the right (wrong?) circumstances. For your teaching wardrobe, choose the heaviest weight fabric that's feasible, and check in the mirror under strong lighting that you aren't showing more than your alignment in a wide-legged forward fold.

Positioning Mats

Early on in your teaching career, you'll cling to your mat like it's a life raft. But there's much to see from every angle of the room, so be on your mat only as much as is needed for you to demonstrate to your students. If you are always in sight, you will remain the focus. Move to the side and your students have to pay attention to their own experience.

It's common for the teacher to set up a mat—or even to have a platform—at the designated front of the room, and the students arranged in rows with the short side of their mats facing the teacher's area. This is also an efficient use of space. When you are in charge of how to set up, you'll need to decide whether to follow this row format, and if you do, which side of the room will be the front. If the room is a narrow rectangle, will you be at the short or the long end of the rectangle? Both of these can make it hard for students to see. Or will students face in to the center of the room, where your mat is set up perpendicular to theirs? In addition to thinking this through, consider the lighting sources in the room.

Also consider the aesthetics of what students are seeing throughout class. Are students looking at you, at a view, or at each other? If the latter, are they familiar to each other, as when you are teaching a team or a corporate class, or are they strangers? My friend Vivian was a high-powered lawyer and, as such, once found herself having yet another stressful day. All day she looked forward to her practice, and she hurried to her Ashtanga Yoga class after work. As is sometimes typical, the class was set up in two rows facing inward toward a central channel. And at the end of this long day, guess who set up across from Vivian: her boss!

Smaller classes and certain formats—like teaching a team or a corporate class at an office, where people know each other—lend themselves to a circle or oval setup. If you do this, be aware that right and left become confusing to people directly across from you. Remind students that you are not mirroring them, or tell them when you are.

Help your students set out their mats in a way that accommodates the needs of the class and your expectation of how full it will be. Be a little bossy up front. Ask students to set their mats close together at the start so that you won't have to disrupt people once class begins. Like choosing the seating arrangement for your dinner guests for the best connections and conversations to occur, where you put students will affect their experience.

In a crowded room, it's good to put taller students in the back. Be aware that students with hearing issues need to be closer to you and may not mention this, so don't be a stickler for bumping tall people to the back of the room.

If you expect a full classroom, it's to everyone's benefit for you to control the way the room fills as it's happening. Decide how many rows there should be, and encourage students to line up in these rows and reasonably close to each other. It may even be helpful to set up some guideline mats, or play the role of sheepdog herding the first few arrivals into the grid you hope to deploy. Some spaces have tape or stickers on the floor to help students align in a tight grid. If there will be a video camera in class, set it up before students enter, and be sure everyone in the shot has signed a model release form.

Expansion is far easier than contraction. If, close to class time, there are empty spaces in the room, then students can move into them. It's far easier to start tight, then spread out, than for each new arrival to cause a reshifting of mats.

If your studio culture and class format allow for students to enter after class has begun, be sure to leave a few obvious holes near the entry door for latecomers' mats. This helps minimize the distraction late arrivals can create. One benefit of online registration is that you can see how many students haven't arrived at the beginning of class, and leave them open spots or even set out mats and props for them.

Feeding Students Off-Site and Online

If teaching a studio class is like hosting a dinner party or running your own restaurant, teaching off-site at a business or private home is like being a caterer. You'll need to think through how to construct your meal without your usual resources on hand. Consider how you will carry props, whether music is feasible, and, for corporate classes, how you might construct a sequence that can be done in office clothes. It's smart to pay a scouting visit ahead of time so you're aware of what the venue offers and what you'll need to supply. For a fascinating look at how real caterers make do in the most unwelcoming venues, read the wonderful book *Hotbox: Inside Catering, the Food World's Riskiest Business*, by Matt and Ted Lee. The brothers evoke a world where the professionals must be present and adapt with flexibility moment to moment—it's a real form of yoga!

If teaching off-site is like being a caterer, recording asynchronous classes for online use or preparing other online content is like working the craft services snack table on a film set. You take great care to prepare and serve food that will suit your audience. But you don't usually get to see how they wind up eating it, since it's being consumed at times that best suit the diners. If you ran craft services, you'd take careful note of what disappears quickly—so you can stock and serve more of that—and what is still untouched at the end of the day. To get the same kind of feedback from your online video viewers, dig in to the statistics. Your video host likely will provide data on views. Even basic hosts like YouTube will give you view counts. More in-depth statistics on how many videos are started, played halfway, or played to completion will be even more useful information. Similarly, if you are posting on social media or a blog, use the insights and statistics available to determine what content is being accessed most often. This will steer you toward what to create next.

Building a Set

If you are setting up for video instead of live class, you'll have a different set of considerations. You'll want a relatively neutral set that reduces visual distraction for viewers and allows them to focus on you. If you are teaching for a studio, they may want a set that clearly identifies the video as part of the studio's brand, with features like a mural or mandala. If you are creating your own content, seek to come up with something attractive but not busy. A plain wall, your mat, and a few plants or pieces of artwork are probably all you'll need. If you're regularly recording, mark where you placed your mat, tripod, and light stands against the floor, so you can recreate the same frame and setup in subsequent videos. Be sure to take some test shots of your sequence before filming, so you can be sure you are well-lit and in the frame throughout the entire video. Be sure to wear clothes that contrast with the background, so you will be most visible.

Props

If you know you'll be using props in your sequence, or simply for convenience to your students, stack a display set of props by your mat. Or carry props over to students as they get settled—it's a warm way to welcome them and make them feel seen. Almost all students benefit from using props, so it's better for them to have props and wind up not using them than to want them and not have them.

To that end, make props a requirement for at least one pose. For example, have students stand on a block (or, for the bigger-footed, two blocks placed short end to short end) for a standing balance pose. Now students see that blocks can make a pose harder—they aren't just to make poses easier. It then is far easier, both physically and psychologically, for them to grab the blocks in a lunge, or in some other pose where they would benefit from using props.

If students still perceive using props as a crutch or an admission that they are not good at yoga, you can change their minds with a little spin: Call props an "upgrade." I've begun doing this for props in savasana. I'll bring a bolster for the knees or a blanket to serve as a pillow and say to the student, "Let me upgrade you."

> ## Nothing Lets Go Unless It Feels Supported
>
> The most profound lesson I received in my own yoga teacher training came in an explanation from Lesa Crocker, my yoga teacher training leader, that "nothing lets go unless it feels supported." Consider a child who receives a glowing report at preschool pickup, Lesa said, but then becomes a holy terror for the rest of the evening. Or imagine you've kept it together during a bad day, but one kind word from your parent or spouse ("Honey, what's wrong?") sets you bawling. Without this compassionate support, the body—especially the muscles and nervous system—will hold tension in. Only in the presence of true support do we feel free to lay our burdens down. As you set up your classroom, and throughout an asana practice with the use of props, be sure to let your students feel the freedom conferred by loving support.

GREET YOUR STUDENTS

Be welcoming to your students. Be ready for them to arrive. Don't be that hostess who's in the shower as her guests show up! Once, I walked into a class at a yoga retreat center five minutes before start time to find the teacher lying on the podium in savasana wrapped in a blanket. I gaped for twenty seconds, then walked right back out and chose a different class.

If you use music, have it settled and set up long before class; don't be messing with your phone, especially with your back to the room, while students come in. Getting soft music rolling can help you calm your own nerves if you're feeling them. When you are nervous, it can be tempting to hide from your students or find busywork. Instead, channel this energy into welcoming students and making them feel comfortable. This will remind you that you are there as a helper, not a performer.

As students arrive, be a gracious host—just like the flight attendant standing by the door. Whenever possible, welcome them individually. Shake hands, learn names, and ask what brings them to yoga. I'll say, "Are you new in town or just new to the studio?" and "Are you new to yoga or just new to us?" Help students get situated: Show them where to leave their shoes, where to put their belongings, where to find the props.

Learning names is easier for some people than for others. Find a graceful way to get refreshers in case you were wrong. (Ask a fellow student discreetly, or simply admit that you feel unsure about the name.) My colleague Alexandra introduced me to this useful prompt: "Hi! Are you a new face for me?" It lets students say, "Yes!" or "I've been a few times but it's been awhile," in which case you follow up with, "Welcome back! Remind me of your name." If you find yourself handling your own class check-in, you'll have a golden chance to learn names: You'll hear it from the student, think it with your brain, and type it into the computer with your hands.

Just as a good host will introduce guests to each other, then drop in a conversation topic or connection and move on, you can foster interpersonal connections in the classroom by introducing your students to each other. This can be especially welcoming to a student who is new in town. Yoga studios can be a powerful site of community connection. People who come to class *want* to be in the presence of other people; otherwise, they'd stream a class at home. Help them feel this connection.

Teachers in Class

If you have the pleasure of having other teachers in class, don't flinch: Rejoice! While your first reaction might be to recoil in horror, thinking you are going to be judged, please reframe your reaction. Unless another teacher is explicitly sent to offer feedback, they are not in your class to evaluate you or to steal from you—they want to be led through a practice and not have to make decisions. As I often put it, they want someone else to drive the bus. Celebrate having teachers as students!

When I have colleagues in class, I make a point of introducing them. This serves a few purposes. First, it cross-promotes their classes. ("This is Alexandra, who teaches the Pilates class before this class. They are wonderful back-to-back! And Alexandra is my regular sub—you'll see her in two weeks when I'm teaching out of town.") Second, it creates a friendly vibe. Students love to know that teachers are students, too, and that the studio community is a supportive one. Third, it gives the teacher permission to practice in her own way without intimidating students. "Oh," they'll think, "she's a teacher, so she's been doing this awhile. I can appreciate the aesthetics of her practice without having to copy it." Sometimes I make this explicit!

Best of all, having teachers in class means you have a group of potential subs who know exactly how you run your classroom and what and how you teach. This is priceless for providing your students continuity when you are away, and thus for best supporting their practices.

When you do have a colleague in class, ask them for feedback. Teachers are always better equipped than students to give you helpful advice. Students will say only, "I liked it!" or "Felt good!" or "That was hard!" Teachers can tell you straight about the clarity of your cuing, the fluidity of your sequences, and the filler words you rely on.

Even with the best-laid plans, every class you teach offers you a new chance to improve. Do you need to tweak the lights, music, tone, volume, or pacing? If something felt off in your last class, it can be helpful to take the time between classes to design new approaches. Was the room too cold? Could you bring a space heater? (Clear it with the building management first!) Was your music not working right? Now's your chance to reflect on your teaching—to troubleshoot until you feel really confident you'll have things the way you want them next time.

SELF-STUDY AND REFLECTION

Much of the development you'll see as a teacher comes incrementally, week to week, as you reflect on your previous class and plan for the next one. Have you heard of a "hostess diary"? It's an old-fashioned device to record a personal debrief after throwing a party. (You can find some cute ones on Amazon or at fancy stationery stores.) The great hostesses make notes after each party. What was the theme or occasion of the party? What was served, who sat where, what was discussed? What could be changed for next time?

The same practice works well for yoga teachers. As soon as is feasible after class, and no later than the next day, take some notes of your own in your journal or notes file. Here's a workbook prompt for you.

Reflect on Class

Make notes on your last class. What did you plan? What went well? What surprised you? Was there any deviation from your plan, and if so, why? How did it land? What did not go well? If it works for you, you can list these as roses (the pros), thorns (the cons), and buds (things to build on next time).

If you wrote out a class plan ahead of time, either on paper or, better yet, on your computer, this could simply be another column or section in the notes, including the date and your reflections on what happened.

SELF-EVALUATION WITH VIDEO

To identify your personal filler words and to quickly clean up your language, I suggest a two-part process, executed every few months. First, record yourself during a real class. This doesn't have to be a professional-grade video; even five minutes captured on your phone will teach you volumes. Be sure you let your students know that you are doing this solely for your self-improvement, and angle the camera so that your students aren't on-screen—or obtain their permission before including them. If you are producing videos—live or edited—regularly watch them for self-evaluation and quality control.

Now take a few deep breaths, settle down, and watch. Here's what to do:

1. Be alone. Watch the video and allow yourself all the cringing you want. If your experience is like mine, you'll think, in quick succession: "Do I really look like that?!?" "Do I really sound like that?!?" and "When did I turn into my mother[/father]?!?"
2. Start over. Look for the good. Pinpoint at least three things you did well.
3. Start over again. Listen for the filler. Hear your go-to words, and determine which could be cut. If you don't hear any, try transcribing your own video, which will likely make them jump out. Even five minutes of typing a transcription will show you what could go. You will very quickly type and see every extraneous word. Even ten minutes of this task will help you immensely.
4. Start over yet again. Use a timer to gauge whether you are offering a similar duration of hold on both sides of asymmetrical poses, and listen to hear whether you give students express permission to stay longer or move out of a pose early.

5. Repeat this exercise, making a new recording and reviewing it, again at regular intervals. Aim to do it a few times each year. It's painful, I know, but self-review with video is one of the quickest tools to make you the best teacher you can be.

Articulate Your Role

If you find your video review disheartening, it can be helpful to articulate what kind of teacher you want to be, so that you have a goal to be striving toward, and to know when you are meeting your vision for yourself as a teacher. Periodic redefinition or reinforcement of your goals will keep you on track.

Start by noting what you think your own teachers do well. Write a little about:

▶ The tone your teachers use with students in class and out of class

▶ The body language and physical reaction your teachers use with students in class and out of class

▶ The interactions you see your teachers use with students in class and out of class, including on social media, if relevant

Now write a description of the kind of teacher you want to be. Notice any friction between how you want to act and how you feel you have been acting.

Consider Your Tone

Given what you know about your students and the content of the class, write a little about the right tone for the class. Is it drill sergeant? Sympathetic coach? Caring mother figure? Sassy best friend? Repeat for each of the classes in your schedule. When you review recordings of your class, be sure to check whether the tone you hear matches the tone you meant to convey.

PEER EVALUATION

Students can't give you the best feedback; they don't have the tools to describe what worked and what didn't. It's like a chef cooking for, say, a teenage lacrosse team—they won't have the palate or vocabulary to critique the food; they're just glad to eat. Your peers, especially your colleagues in teacher training and at the venue where you teach, will be better. To get useful feedback, the chef must serve other chefs and experienced eaters. And it's probably best if these chefs are skilled in the same kind of cooking—that is, your best evaluators will come from a similar background as you and work with a student population similar to yours.

Invite a friend to class expressly for this evaluation. If your friend can set up discreetly in the back, they may even make a few notes. If the venue allows observation and you are especially open and willing to succeed, you can have them sit and watch instead of participating, or record a whole class for them to review. (At Carolina Yoga, we do not allow nonparticipating students to sit and observe class, as we think it creates a strange situation for the participating students.) If you are teaching in video format, share your recordings with a colleague to get feedback.

BE KIND TO YOURSELF

Growth is hard. Growth requires being uncomfortable. But without opening yourself up to constructive criticism, there will be no growth at all, and your career will wither on the vine. All your good intentions about helping your students through yoga will come to nothing if you don't challenge yourself to improve.

When it's tough to hear a critique, go back to the start. Remember why you love yoga and why you became a teacher. It may be useful to revisit the work you did in part 1 of this book. And remember this quote from Winston Churchill: "I am always ready to learn, although I do not always like being taught." The improvement is worth the discomfort.

Pep Talk and Rainy Day Notes

Give yourself a pep talk! Using the voice of a loving friend, write yourself a blurb about all your good points as a teacher. If you like, distill it into a phrase ("You're authentic!") or a word ("Real!") that you can revisit as needed.

In a notes file or a journal, collect praise you've received from your students, and visit these rainy-day notes to cheer yourself up when you are feeling disheartened or down.

ENTHUSIASTIC STUDENTSHIP

Take classes with a teacher's ear—listen for what works and what doesn't. Stay attuned to the choices, conscious and unconscious, that your teachers make when you are in the classroom. Feel your way through transitions that are useful; notice how it feels and how the room looks when something doesn't land. Set up in different parts of the room to see what the student experience is like there. The view from the back and the front could be vastly different; being closer to the door or window or farther from it may affect the student experience a lot.

It's especially useful to be a student in the very classroom(s) where you teach, so you can notice things that you won't see when you're teaching. Strive to have the same experience your students have, down to using the studio-issued mat. You may find that your hands slip in downward-facing dog or your knees need some extra cushioning in tabletop, and these observations can translate into a direct positive experience for your students when you offer modifications in your next class.

Make note of anything that works particularly well, and consider how you would do things differently when things don't work well. It can help to put this down on paper. For example, my don'ts would be having the music too quiet (I find this a distraction), shining bright light in students' eyes, and not telling students what to expect in the course of the class.

> ### Classroom Management
>
> Describe your ideal classroom environment from the point of view of both a student and a teacher. List any don'ts you've personally witnessed, and make notes about how you would do things differently.

BE A TEACHING ASSISTANT

Once you are comfortable offering manual assists, or even just quiet verbal cuing and demonstrating in a large beginner class, offer to assist in a friend's class, or your primary teacher's class. This affords you a chance to look at what's happening at some remove.

You can observe the teacher without needing to follow their cues, which gives you insight into language, energy, tone, and pacing. You can see which cues land and which don't. You can also observe the students as a whole and as individuals without being in charge of the entire room at once.

After each class you assist, make notes as you would for your own class. List the sequence and, if relevant, the theme; detail who was in the room; note roses, thorns, and buds.

LOOK AT MODELS

Find master teachers online. If there is a class you especially enjoyed participating in as a student, watch it again as an observer, without participating. What makes it special? Is it the teacher's sequencing, cuing, pacing, language? Reverse engineer the parts you like best to discover ways you can deploy the magic in your own classes. The humorist Finley Peter Dunne wrote that it is the duty of newspapers to "comfort the afflicted and afflict the comfortable." I would apply this in a serious way to yoga teachers. I've learned a lot from watching Leslie Kaminoff, who fulfills the role of comforting the afflicted by reassuring students when they are confused and afflicting the comfortable by challenging those who would benefit from it.

When one class ends, the reflection begins, as does the planning for the next one. Now you're ready to lead the next class through a yoga practice! That's our focus in chapter 8.

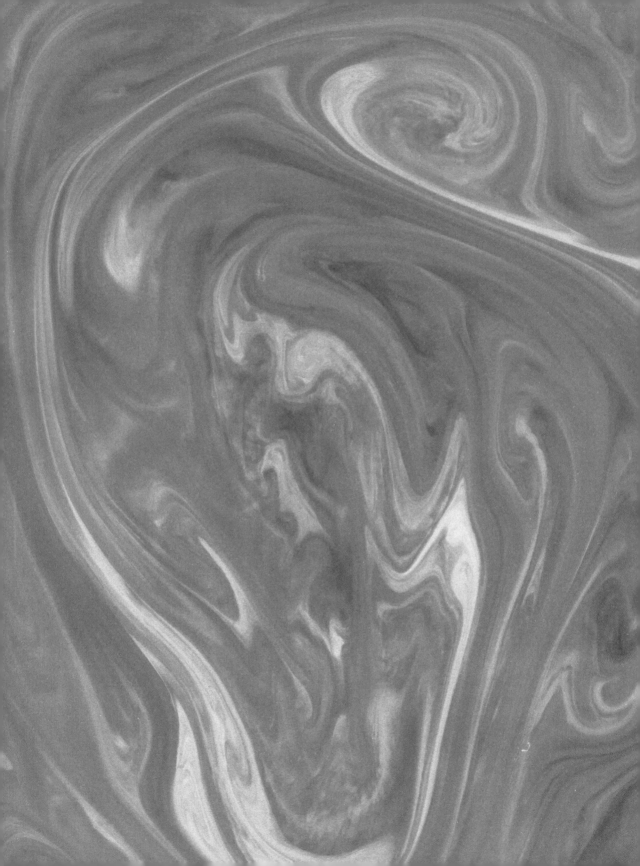

8

Nailing It: Executing Your Plans in Class

· ·

HERE, WE ARE concerned more with *how* you teach your class than *what* you teach. As the saying goes, people will forget what you did, they will forget what you said, but they will remember how you made them feel. Perfecting your presentation in the categories below will leave your students feeling good. If you've been teaching for a while, you may have fallen into habits that create a less-than-ideal tone in the room. Paying attention to your *hows* now that you are comfortable with your *whats* will help you be a better teacher.

As a yoga teacher, when you take a class as a student your attention is naturally drawn to the poses and the sequencing. But for the majority of your students, the quality of the experience matters far more than the exact pose routine. In your next several class experiences as a student, focus on the delivery rather than the package, on the container more than the content, on the service rather than the dish. Then make a list of what your favorite teachers do during class to create the best experience. Here's what I think a good teacher does.

ESTABLISH EXPECTATIONS AND FULFILL THEM

Attending yoga for the first time—or taking a class with a new teacher or in a new studio—can be incredibly intimidating to students. By intentionally creating a welcoming environment, you'll ensure that students have a positive experience that leaves them open to yoga's benefits and eager to return.

The welcome and introduction you give in the first few minutes of class are like the greeting and instructions your flight attendant announces as your plane taxis to the runway for takeoff. For those new to class—the nervous flyers, in this analogy—this is an opportunity to receive important safety information and orientation to the space. And while frequent flyers may tune out the seat belt fitting and emergency landing instructions, hearing the familiar spiel gives them a cue to wrap up what they were doing, put their electronics in airplane mode, and prepare for the transition to flight. If you are producing a series of video classes, having the same title card or short intro clip leading in to each one serves as a visual cue to frame the class.

As you prepare your welcoming remarks, remember the five Ws and the one H: who, what, when, where, why, and how. Briefly cover these at the start of class to give students a clear picture of where the class is going and how to find and use the tools to care for their needs.

Who

As you begin the class proper, even in a class full of regulars, it's polite to introduce yourself. *Say your name!* If you are subbing a class, share a few words about your teaching background so that students have some context for their upcoming experience. But don't apologize for being a sub—remember, you're not Bryan. Be yourself.

What and When

In preflight announcements, flight attendants mention the flight number, destination, and flying time. Do the same for your students. Tell them the class name (especially when there's another class with a similar start time, or if there's a chance they could be in the wrong room!). Give a broad overview of the class intensity. Be sure to say what time class will end, which holds you accountable for ending on time and wards off student frustration that can occur when the end time is unclear. It's also helpful to confirm end time when you are subbing a class.

Example—who, what, and when: "Welcome! I'm Sage Rountree—and yes, that is my real name, though it sounds like a yoga handle. This is a seventy-five-minute Yoga for Athletic Balance class; we'll end with a nice, long relaxation period and wrap up at 7:15.

My presumption is that you've already gotten in a workout for the day, or you're taking a rest day today, so we'll keep things simple and low to the ground to help you balance the work you do in training."

Where

Invite your students to take a moment to orient themselves, finding exits, restrooms, and props. Taking the time to explain the physical layout of the space encourages students to take care of their own needs during class, breaking for water or picking up props.

Example—where: "If you need a break during class, please use this door. The bathrooms and water fountain are just outside. Props are along this wall. Help yourself to them now or at any time, as they can really enhance your experience."

Why

Why have you chosen the sequence of the class? What effects will the poses have? Do they build strength? Flexibility? Balance? Beyond the physical, why are we doing yoga? Explain these reasons to your students briefly at the beginning, and return to the reasons as class unfolds.

Example—why: "As athletes, we develop sport-specific strengths. The shadow side to this are sport-specific weaknesses. In tonight's class, we'll investigate where these imbalances may hide in our bodies by comparing the experience in standing poses on one side with the experience on the other. This will show us where we can shore up our weaknesses to greater apply our strengths, and this goes for the breath and mind as much as for the body."

How

What is the mood of class? Is there an attitude students should cultivate? Are we approaching the poses with courage, holding them longer to build strength? Are we looking instead to soften and relax? Set the tone for your class by encouraging students to set an intention around how they will be in the practice.

Example—how: "As we observe the less-strong parts of our bodies, we might feel surprise, frustration, or a strong urge to fix things right away. And as we notice the parts that are strong, we might feel relief or pride. When these feelings arise, let's notice them objectively. This teaches us equanimity, the ability to maintain center in the face of shifting circumstances."

All told, your welcoming remarks won't take very long—the combined examples above take under ninety seconds to read aloud—but they will have a major impact on the students' experience. They will establish the expectations you will fulfill throughout the class.

Write Out Your Opening Remarks

Take the time to write out your standard opening spiel. If you don't have one yet, cover the five Ws and one H in your draft. If you do have one, challenge yourself to find new language to convey the same information. Being able to do that will help you feel fresh week to week and will keep your students engaged with the right balance of consistent information in a varied package.

CREATE CONNECTION

One definition of *yoga*, union, is connection. Students come to class because they want to feel connected, both intrapersonally—in mind, body, breath, and spirit—and also interpersonally—with the teacher, with the community, with others.

Make Eye Contact

Following the steps in chapter 7 to prepare for class will set the stage for connection. During the class itself, be sure to connect with your students by looking them in the eye. I know: Eye contact can be intimidating and difficult, especially when you're also looking at students' bodies for safe alignment and to be sure that your cues are landing. But your students came to class for connection. They want to be seen.

Challenge yourself to make regular eye contact with each of your students and to smile as you do. Of course you are looking at their bodies to be sure your cues land and they are out of danger of hurting themselves, but also look above the neck to their faces. (Imagine your student chastising you: "My eyes are up here!") This can be very hard, particularly for shy teachers, but practice goes a long way to upping your comfort level. You might set yourself the goal of making eye contact with everyone in the room at least once during the movement practice, or looking one person in the eye in every standing pose. If this is difficult, practice with your peers, friends, and family, until it grows more comfortable. Less than one second of eye contact with a smile goes a very long way in the yoga classroom.

In Carolina Yoga Company's teacher training, we get trainees in front of the class immediately so they can begin getting used to the eyes on them. If you've already been in front of the classroom, you know that adapting to being seen like this is critical for your ability to lead the class with confidence.

When you are teaching a video class where it's only you talking on camera, looking directly at the camera lens is the equivalent of making eye contact during conversation. Look at the camera frequently, with a smile—it's far more engaging to the viewer than to completely disregard the camera. If you are teaching a virtual private lesson or a group class in real time, it's tempting to look at the screen displaying your students more than at the camera—but be sure you look at the camera, so your viewers can feel a sense of connection. On the other hand, if you are video-recording a demonstration but adding voice-over later, eye contact seems out of place. Self-review will teach you what works best.

Challenge Yourself

In your next few classes, set yourself the goal of making eye contact with every student at least once. Notice what this requires: You may need to move around the room more, or work to catch one student's eye. Make some notes about how this felt and what, if anything, made it difficult.

Assists

Writ large, your entire class is an assist to your students: You help them find connection between mind, body, and breath. Your clear cueing offers a verbal assist, and your demonstrations offer a visual assist. Beyond these, you may choose to offer physical assists. These can be and have been the subject of whole books on their own, but they are best learned in person from an experienced teacher and practiced on other teachers until you feel extremely clear and comfortable with the how and why of giving every single assist. Because this is a broad topic for you to study in person over several months, years, or decades, I'll make only a few comments on the subject here, keyed to how to handle the whole room of students rather than exactly what to administer to any individual.

First, make it explicitly clear to students that they can always decline an assist, pose to pose, moment to moment. You should have explicit consent before laying hands on a student. Better yet, have each person in your class choose whether to opt in to receiving assists. A cheap way to do this is to buy a deck of cards and give one to each student, who can then place it at the front of their mat. When the face is up, a student is open to receiving assists; when the face is down, they are asking not to be touched. Point out to the whole class that they are welcome to flip their cards at any point, with no explanation needed, and they may turn it over many times during class. This gives room for people who have, say, a knee injury to avoid any imposed outside stress on the joint in standing poses but still receive the benefits of a savasana assist. And students who are touch-averse can, with very little effort, quietly signal that they decline any physical assist.

Let your students know the nature of your manual assists, as well as your verbal corrections. Are they corrections for safety? (Check yourself: Are they corrections for aesthetics, to bring the shape into alignment with your Platonic ideal for it? Or are they useful for students? Aesthetic corrections are useful in a photo shoot but confusing for students in class.) Are they ways for the students to gain more awareness of their bodies in the shape, perhaps by cuing the movement of energy? Are they encouragements to relax more? Gentle congratulatory pats on the back? When your touch is put in context, students can make an informed decision about whether to receive or not. You can explain as part of your ask for consent: "May I stabilize your hips with my hands to help you balance?" "Is it OK to put my hands on your arms here to free up space for your shoulders? Does that feel better or worse?"

One school of thought is to assist on an ad-hoc basis, offering assists—verbal, visual, or touch—to those who appear to need them, especially if they are holding a pose in a way that could invite injury, or if you see a way to create more ease. This triage can be really important, giving the most attention to the students who need it. If you offer assists case by case, be aware that it implies that your assists are correcting something the students have done wrong. Cumulatively, this can cause students to worry about how they are messing up when they receive an assist. For some personalities, it's gratifying to learn how to do things the "right" way; for other personalities, it's disheartening to always feel "wrong." (Your thinking here should align with your sense of the rules you articulated in part 1.)

Another approach to manual assists is to work through the entire room systematically, mat by mat. Each touch might last for only one or two breaths, which makes this an appealing addition to a flow yoga class for those who like being touched. It also removes the sense of value judgment from the touch, because it's clear to the students that everyone gets a turn to receive and it's obvious when it's their turn. If you take this approach, take note when you reach asymmetrical poses. It's especially gratifying for students when you can catch everybody in order again on the second side, so that they receive the same assist on both the left and the right. If this is how you work, consent cards can keep the pacing fluid.

HOLD THE SPACE

"Holding the space" is a term we like in yoga—it is another way to describe creating a safe container for your students to have connection. You'll have already made choices about the container before and as your students arrive. During class, here's how you can best hold the space.

Offer Appropriate Demonstrations

Depending on the experience level of your students, they may need a lot of demonstration on your part to understand what you are guiding them to do. In a class with more experienced students—or even just some experienced students situated in everyone's sight line—teacher demonstration is less necessary.

Don't overdemonstrate. Hold the demo just long enough to make your point. This can be really tough for new teachers. Remember, you're leading yoga, not doing your own practice. While some forms of group exercise—step aerobics, Spinning—and most video classes do better with the teacher participating with the student, in most forms of live or real-time yoga, the teacher simply leads and watches the students. Imagine going to a restorative yoga class and having the teacher take each pose! Differentiate between your own practice and your teaching in service of the students.

Exceptions include certain cases where the students would resent the teacher blithely saying, "You've got this, just five more breaths," while not participating. Our Pilates classes at Carolina Yoga Company work like that, and for the most part, it's how I teach yin yoga too. In these modalities, practicing alongside students gives me a sense of how many reps to do or how the pose is unfolding over time, and it avoids fostering student resentment toward the teacher. Even in a class where you offer minimal demonstration, it's smart to join your students for boat pose, for example, which doesn't require much warm-up.

Some studios offer "led" yoga classes, which means the teacher is on their mat alongside the students. The teacher cues as they go along, while taking each pose. Though the word "led" may be confusing, and is not to be conflated with Ashtanga's Led Primary Series, a set sequence that contains the same poses every time, the intention is clear: It's a more collegial, participatory class, and together the teacher and students can journey toward more complex asanas as they have warmed up to them as a group.

One benefit of not demonstrating is that you will have more time to observe your students, and you won't get in the odd position of talking through your armpit in child's pose or turning your back to students for extended periods of time. If you need to show such a pose, do it for only a moment. And consider the best view for students to understand what you are asking for them—you may need to turn, or to move to a different side of the room.

In some poses, a demonstration is useful before students begin to move into the shape. This goes for all inversions, for many prone poses, and for some supine poses, like bridge, where it's not easy or even safe to try to turn and see what's happening. In these instances, ask the students to stop, stand if necessary so they can see you, and offer a quick demo. Sometimes you need to be firm in your instruction: "Even if you are used to shoulder stand, please stop and watch this setup before coming into the shape today."

Your students learn in different ways. Some are fine with verbal cues only; others are visual learners and need to see what you're doing before they do it themselves. You'll quickly recognize the visual learners in class: When you raise your arm to tuck your hair behind your ear, their arms will lift, too! These mirror movements give you insight into your own physical tics and nervous habits. So will watching a video recording of your class, as discussed in the previous chapter.

Corals, Sharks, and Fish

Beyond your demonstrations, balance stillness and movement in the classroom. Don't be like a coral, fixed in place, rooted, unmoving. This bores your students and keeps them from feeling seen and therefore from feeling safe and supported. It can also ignore students situated in areas of the room that you can't see well or from where they can't see you.

At the same time, don't be like a shark, constantly circling through the room. This makes your students nervous, especially if you are a heavy walker stomping through the room in continual movement. In a crowded room, those of us who like to move can wind up pacing back and forth at the front like a caged tiger or a bad stage actor. This is also unnerving for your students.

Instead, be like a fish: Move some, pause some. Take your time to move slowly and lightly through the room and to pause in different areas. You'll see a lot more when you move through the room than you would clinging to the life raft of your mat.

As you move like a fish, read the currents of the room. When students are moving, move; when students are still, be still or move gently and slowly. When students are balancing, don't distract them by moving—unless you're purposefully *trying* to make it tougher to balance. In fact, consider cuing balance poses from out of students' sight lines. Or, if you are at the front of the room to demonstrate, try dropping into a squat once you've given your demo.

If you aren't going to demo, you can still use your hands as if conducting a symphony. Don't just stand there with your hands folded; find something to do with your arms. Let them describe the energetics of the pose, raise a finger to indicate an upcoming change to the sequence, point to areas in your body where students might feel the work of the poses. Apart from being visually interesting, this is useful for students with hearing problems.

Be aware of the dynamic of your placement relative to the students. In general, aim to stay one level higher than your class. Don't lie down except for quick visual demonstrations. When students are low on the mat, particularly in a pose like happy baby, don't loom over them; sit down or kneel. Conversely, don't sit low on your mat while students are standing and active. Exception: dropping out of students' line of sight in a balance pose to avoid disrupting their *drishti*. Also, if you are injured and need to teach while seated, do! It's almost always better to teach than to get a substitute, unless you are contagious.

When you are teaching on video, of course, things are different. You may never leave your mat for the entire class, as you demonstrate along the way. Or, you may have one or more students demonstrate while you guide; but you'll still need to stay in the frame, so you won't move much. With recorded video, you may have a videographer either operate the main camera or use a second one to get B-roll that will then be edited in. This B-roll could track you through the room or focus on different students in the context of the practice, as the lesson demands.

Make Space

If your students wear glasses, it can be relaxing for them to remove them during savasana, or necessary for them to come off for inversions or downward-facing dog. In these cases, encourage your students to rest their glasses on top of a yoga block so that you don't inadvertently step on them when you move through the room. Similarly, you may want to encourage students to keep only the important items—props, a water bottle, a second layer and no other personal items—by them on the mat, so you have some space to move through the room.

Mirroring

Mirroring is the act of reversing right and left when you face your students, so that when you move your left arm, you say "right," and the students move their right arms. This is an important skill to develop, especially when teaching on video. It definitely takes some getting used to—I'm still working on it after almost two decades! Because of the steep learning curve for offering mirrored cues, you might choose not to mirror during the early stage of your career. If that's your choice, you could take one of these approaches:

Turn sideways. For lunges and other poses that stagger one foot forward and the other foot back, a side view can be very useful. This allows you to say "right" and do "right" at the same time your students do. Be careful, though, not to turn your back on students for long. If you're doing a reverse triangle or a twisting lunge, for example, change sides on the mat so that you can see your students. Or turn to face them or the camera. Putting two mats in a cross will give you traction for these demos, if needed; you could also do without a mat entirely.

Use landmarks, not directions. This is a great workaround not only for mirroring but also for those of us who get left and right confused even on good days. Instead of saying, "Lean to your left," choose a landmark in the room or on your set and say, "Lean toward the window," or "the door," or "the brick wall," or whatever is an obvious direction. This approach helps you grow more comfortable mirroring, without needing to flip left and right in your head.

Reference letters. I once taught a workshop in a gym where someone had taped a giant letter R on the top left corner of the back wall, and a giant letter L on the top right corner. Brilliant! This is an easy addition behind the camera, when you are recording video. I've seen teachers draw R and L or use R and L stickers along the edges of their mats to help them call out the mirror directions.

USE REFINED, EFFICIENT LANGUAGE
Speak Clearly in Second-Person Singular Imperative

Different schools, styles, and programs will teach different principles for clear language in class. At Kripalu, for example, the preferred article is "the," not "your": "Lift the right leg," not "Lift your right leg." And in the YogaFit style, there is a preference for gerunds: "Lifting your arms, lowering your torso." There are arguments for these choices, and if you find them most natural or your studio or lineage subscribes to them, please keep going.

I speak to my students in the second-person singular, as it sounds most natural to me. Grammatically, the subject "you" is implied; you'll issue a verb, with the object as a body part. "[You] inhale and lift your arms." Thus the class becomes a conversation between you and each individual student. This is not to imply you can't or shouldn't say, "Let's all come to standing." Using the first person-plural *we* a few times shows that we are all in this together.

Even in a room full of students, each student experiences your directions discretely as an individual. Strive to forge a connection between you and each listener. To that end, your language should comprise complete sentences in a one-to-one second-person singular conversation with the student. Say, "Lift your right leg," not "Lift your right legs," not "Lift the right leg," not "Lift that right leg," not "Lift our right leg" (sure, *yoga* means union, but do we all have one collective leg?!?), not "Lift our right legs," and not "Lifting your right leg," unless that is directly followed by an action verb: "Lifting your right leg, try to keep your right hip point facing down."

The second-person singular means you are talking directly to one person. And do it in the imperative: "Lift your leg," not "lifting our legs." When we string together *-ing* words without a command, students never get to hear a complete sentence. Compare "Lifting your arms, lowering them to your thighs, inhaling, arching your back, exhaling, rounding your back" with "Lift your arms. Lower them to your thighs. Inhale and arch your back. Exhale and round your back." The latter is more direct and contains complete sentences. This is much more satisfying for your listeners.

Close the Loop

If you are teaching a flow class that links breath and movement, first cue breath, then cue movement. ("Inhale, lift your arms overhead. Exhale, fold forward.") In these cases, be sure you close the loop of the cue: Don't say *inhale* without issuing a matching *exhale* cue. I once realized I'd left students hanging when someone gasped, "Can we exhale?"

Work from the Ground Up

In a physical description of a pose, start from the ground—the feet, hands and feet, or whatever is in contact with the mat. From this base, choose another one, two, or three actions for students to take or areas for them to be aware of. More than three or four cues in any shape is too many for students to process, especially if you are teaching a movement-based class.

Season to Taste with Figurative Language

Depending on what comes naturally to you and what fits with the student population and studio vibe, you may enjoy sprinkling figurative language through your cuing. I rely a lot on food analogies, especially the terms "spicy" and "sweet," rather than "hard" and "easy" or "more" and "less." But I also draw spontaneously on topical analogies, and when I am teaching a group with a common interest—a basketball team, for example—I draw on analogies between the movements of the poses and their movement on the court, as well as comparing the focus and presence we need on the mat to what we need in the game.

Use your figurative language wisely. Don't say "press your palms into the earth" when you really mean "press your palms into the mat." If you're going to use figurative language, really go for it: "Press your palms down as though you are shooting roots deep into the earth." If this kind of language isn't natural to you, don't use it! Your students will be drawn to you precisely because you're being your authentic self. Don't cloak yourself in flowery words if it feels weird.

Cut the Filler

Much of what you'll say in class can be cut. Consider these filler words and phrases.

- ▶ And now
- ▶ From here
- ▶ We're gonna/we're going to
- ▶ So
- ▶ Actually

Usually these and similar phrases can simply be cut, with nothing to replace them. If you need to cue that something different is about to happen, say, "We're changing things this round," "Listen closely," "*This* time," "Key change," or "Plot twist!" These give students a heads-up without being useless filler, words that are so overused that they've lost their ability to grab students' attention.

"Just" is a special favorite of yoga teachers. It makes the instruction sound simple, easy, doable: "Just breathe." OK, great. But don't overuse "just"! It can diminish your stature, and perhaps that's subconsciously what you're trying to do: to make yourself smaller. Don't! Your students need you to be big—the world needs you to be big.

"Nice" is another low-value word. "Take a nice deep breath" doesn't mean much, nor does "Feel a nice big stretch." Instead, be specific: "Take a deep breath that you feel expanding your torso in all directions." "You may feel this as a hamstring stretch along the backs of your thighs, but back off if you feel it in your knees or at your sitting bones."

Often these filler words disappear when you take your own deep breaths and slow down the pacing of your speech—they were simply space holders. Remember that it's not only fine, it's really good to have quiet periods in class.

Close the Thesaurus

While you're self-editing and cutting out the filler words, know that at the other end of the spectrum, you may be using some fancy words—I call them five-dollar words—too much as well. These evocative words carry a big punch when you use them. And they are really useful, but only when deployed once per class. The problem comes when you start to rely on the word and use it multiple times in one class, at which point it quickly draws attention to itself. Think of words like *unravel*, *slice*, or *float*. Each of these highlights an action you want your students to take or feel. But after one use, replace them with *unwind*, *reach*, or *lift*. These one-dollar words are more digestible for students.

Similarly, here are some lovely phrases that work well in small doses but grow distracting in bigger servings:

I want you to. Once or twice in a class, in the context of "I want you to feel this here," or "I want you to modify to your own tastes," "I want you to" can be a useful and powerful phrase. When overdeployed, it draws the student out of inner experience and into the narrative of what *you* want. This can encourage students to do things simply to please you; alternatively, it can make them grumpy ("Why is it all about you?").

I invite you to. In trauma-informed yoga, all instructions are invitations. This creates a student-directed environment where the teacher is making suggestions, not commands. But this can be conveyed in a few sentences at the start of class and referred to a few times during class. There's no need to start every instruction with "I invite you to."

Please. Similarly, using "please" a few times goes a long way. Too many make you sound needy. One "please step to the front of your mat" or "please come to table pose" is enough.

Edit yourself ruthlessly, and seek specificity over vagueness. You'll sound more professional, your students will hear you more clearly, and everyone will benefit.

Embrace the Quiet

You aren't being paid by the word. Don't fear silence; embrace it. Teaching yoga in a classroom is not like delivering stand-up, announcing the news on the radio, or giving a talk at the United Nations. There's no such thing as dead air, and it's OK to be silent. When you don't know what to say, say nothing!

When you *do* know what to say, give time for your students to process it. Constantly aim for more silence, less talking. You'll recognize experienced teachers because they are good at keeping their mouths shut. They know just what to say to get students safely into and out of the poses, as well as what to say to direct their attention during poses. The rest of the time, they allow for silence.

Silence can be an asset to you as a new teacher. Let go of the need to fill the room with the constant sound of your voice, and let students go into inner experience. The more nervous, anxious, or unsure you feel, the more quiet time you should allot in class. Give your students enough direction (one or two cues) to get into a posture or a breath exercise, then zip it and let them be there. If you see them getting antsy, drop in a cue to turn attention to breath, to stay present, or to relax, and again grow quiet. Too much talking creates the very opposite effect from what's intended: a sense of clarity and connection.

A major exception to this rule: When you are teaching online classes, especially live classes, where slow Internet speeds can affect student experience, big chunks of silence can make students worry that the video has stalled. In these situations, preface the silence: "We'll be holding this yin yoga pose for three minutes, and I'll get quiet except for a few check-ins to remind you we're still here together." Then every twenty or thirty seconds, give a quick cue: "Where could you relax more?" "Stay with your breath." "We're still here."

Volume and Pacing

Find the right pace and volume for the class. The majority of new teachers need to slow down and speak up. When you're excited, it's easy to talk too fast. To help yourself talk more slowly, borrow this tip I learned early on as a radio announcer: Try tapping your foot very slowly. That should slow your pacing.

That said, you don't want to talk so slowly that you're dragging down the mood of the class or affecting a "yoga voice," nor would you want to be yelling at your students. If your cues aren't landing, you may need to offer them louder. If your students are cringing, tone it down. Ask a friend or a regular student to signal if you are too quiet or too loud, or self-review with an audio or video recording of your teaching, as discussed in chapter 7.

There's a big difference between a calm voice and a quiet voice. Speaking too quietly will frustrate your students. So will drawing out words in an unnatural lilt, or hissing *ssssse*s in a misguided attempt to slow your speech. Your voice in class should be very similar to your voice in natural conversation. Don't get singsongy or more airy-fairy than you are naturally. Reviewing a recording will help you find the places where your teaching voice differs from your everyday voice. If you're not sure what your everyday voice is, record yourself having dinner with your family or a conversation with a friend, then compare that to a recording of yourself in class.

Cleaning up your language is tough. Often, once you identify a problem phrase or tone, it gets worse before it gets better. In teacher training, when we point out an overused phrase during one student's practice teaching, we often find that it suddenly infects the entire room of trainees. This is part of the process; don't sweat it too much.

Sanskrit

Depending on the culture of your studio, Sanskrit may be an integral part of students' and your managers' expectations. Using Sanskrit can connect the modern yoga practice to its roots. You might be using Sanskrit for pose names (ideally, followed immediately by their common English names) or for chanting.

If your studio culture is not Sanskrit-heavy, and if your class doesn't have many foreign-language speakers coming through, you can probably go without it. While the idea of Sanskrit as a common language among yogis is nice, some schools give different names to the same poses; there are pronunciation differences among schools and teachers; and using Sanskrit can come off as cultural appropriation. When you're a new teacher, in particular, wedging in Sanskrit with passable pronunciation is one more thing to stress over; going without frees you to focus your energy on what your students need.

I find myself using almost no Sanskrit, with the one exception of using "savasana" instead of saying "corpse pose." This could be an expression of aversion to the imagery of a dead body. The sutras would classify this as *abhinivesha*, fear of death, and categorize it as one of the *kleshas*, or obstacles to achieving liberation. But I think I use it in an attempt to convey that the final relaxation pose at the end of class can be done supine, prone, side lying, or propped up. And I do always end with *namaste*.

ESTABLISH TIMING THAT FEELS GOOD

Here's a true confession from most yoga teachers: We always go faster on the second side. This happens for a variety of reasons, prime among them that we have said all our best cues on the first side and haven't grown comfortable with silence, or that we have mismanaged time and see the clock ticking. Once you recognize these common reasons, you can begin to correct them.

Too many words. Don't recite a laundry list of everything you have to say about a pose at its introduction. Instead, save some of your cues for the second side or the next round. Give no more than three instructions on the first side or instance of a pose. If they land well, students won't need much direction on the second side. This frees you to be quiet, to add some metaphorical or figurative language, or to point back to the theme you introduced at the start of class as you reach the second side.

Unawareness. Use a watch, or keep your eye on the clock. It's easy with a little practice. Leave room for students to stay a little longer than your cuing or to move out of a pose sooner than the official cue comes. One way to do this is to slot in a neutral or symmetrical pose after every long-held asymmetrical pose. For example, follow a reclining twist with a cobbler pose or a bent-knee savasana, then lead the twist on the other side and remind students that they know their bodies best and thus will know best when to move back to neutral.

Record your class, and you'll quickly see where the second side doesn't get its due. The timer doesn't lie.

"The Cook Must Simply Grin and Bear It"

Don't apologize too much for your mistakes in cuing class. This draws attention to things your students likely won't even notice you messed up. While a quick, "Whoops, I forgot triangle pose," or "Sorry, I mean your left leg!" demonstrates your humanity and can get the class all on the same page, be careful not to overapologize. Only you know exactly where your sequences are heading; your students don't know all the things you meant to say. In an August 20, 2004, *New York Times* opinion piece, Chef Alex Prud'homme said of his mentor Julia Child, "If a dish goes horribly wrong, like a 'vile' eggs Florentine she once made for a friend, Julia instructed, 'Never apologize.' She considered it unseemly for a cook to twist herself into knots of excuses and explanations. Such admissions 'only make a bad situation worse,' she said, by drawing attention to one's shortcomings (or self-perceived shortcomings) and prompting your guest to think: Yes, you're right, this really is an awful meal. 'The cook must simply grin and bear it.'"

OFFER A QUALITY SAVASANA

Just as a delicious dessert can rescue a dinner party whose main course was burned, a great savasana experience will leave students feeling satisfied. Don't scrimp on it!

It takes self-discipline, nothing more, to leave enough time for savasana. Exert this self-discipline. Know how long your closing remarks take and how long you'd like to have students in savasana. Work back from there.

Aim for savasana to take about 10 percent of the class time. Thus, allot six minutes in a sixty-minute class, seven or eight in a seventy-five-minute class, and nine minutes in a ninety-minute class. As you know from your own student experience, a too-short stay in savasana isn't relaxing, while staying too long in the pose can either leave you groggy or, if relaxation is elusive, agitate you. You want students to really settle but not fall asleep. Sometimes, it feels like there's a moment when the whole room sinks into relaxation. Let them linger for a minute or two beyond that point, then walk them back out.

Before beginning savasana, preview what will happen. Offer to deliver props, mention whether you will be assisting (if it's a big room and you won't have time to make it but students are used to having assists, encourage them to do a self-assist by smoothing their foreheads and lengthening their necks), mention whether there will be music, and give a sense of how long the period will last and what will mark its end. While most classes end with the teacher talking the students out of savasana to finish seated, some styles of yoga—hot yoga especially—leave students to take savasana to taste, in which case the teacher says *namaste*, then leaves the room as the class settles in. Know that your students who come from a hot yoga background might be expecting the latter.

If you are teaching via video, end class by putting people in savasana and either encouraging them to stay as long as they like (as done in some hot yoga styles) or telling them how long the savasana will last (then, at the end of your timed period, you can again encourage students to linger in savasana, if they have the time and inclination). Either way, you and your students should be sure to check that the host service is not set to auto-play another video when yours ends!

Because of the relaxation shift that happens in savasana, there's a point beyond which it's too late to touch students—maybe around 60 percent of the time held. If you will be offering assists, know how long your go-to assists take, and don't start if you can't do the whole room.

I used to always make a point that students can opt out of savasana assists, by saying something like, "I'll be coming around with a shoulder press, neck pull, and short head rub to help you settle. If you're not in the mood, growl or shake your head when you hear me approach, and I'll pass you by." An opt-out has happened to me exactly twice in seventeen years of teaching—and once it was the student I knew best in the room, who demurred, saying, "I'm too sweaty!" Often, teachers will say, "Place a hand on your belly if you don't want an assist here." But that penalizes the no-thanks crowd by sticking them with a hand on the belly—when do they know that they can move it? Must they spend all of savasana with a lopsided arm?

Now I prefer an opt-in model. Ask for people to put their hands on their belly if they *do* want an assist. This is especially useful for keeping track of who's already been touched, especially if you have a helper or are assisting in another teacher's class. This language should be friendly and nonjudgmental: "I'll be coming around to offer a shoulder press and neck pull, and I'll have lavender oil on my arm so you can smell it without it getting transferred to you. If this sounds good to you, please put a hand on your belly now, and you can move it when I arrive to assist you."

A slow, unhurried trip out of savasana seals in its benefits and sets up your students for a sweet end to class. Take your time coming out. If you have a chime, use it. I like to preview the sound as students are settling in, with a statement like, "Near the end of this period, I'll sound this chime. Between now and then, there's nothing you need to do or make happen but rest and breathe." That way, the sound becomes a bookmark for the resting period. You can then walk students out by having them first connect with their breath, next begin to move their bodies, then finally turn to one side and sit up.

Why the Right Side?

You may have noticed that many teachers roll students to the right side to rest on the way from savasana to sitting. (In prenatal yoga, students are told to roll to the left, to take pressure off the vena cava.) Some people will talk about balancing the energies in the body or facing toward the sun. My take is far more mundane: It's a classroom management tool to orient everyone in an orderly fashion. When students don't know each other, it can be alarming to blink eyes open and lock gazes immediately with a stranger lying close by. If you have a group who know each other, or there's enough room, allow students to choose either side, which the folks with shoulder or hip issues will especially appreciate.

CLOSE WITH GRACE

Once students are sitting, you'll move through the closing part of class. You don't have to follow each of the steps outlined below. Include the elements that come to you naturally. If you don't feel comfortable chanting, don't chant; students will register your discomfort. Think of the progression below like the liturgical elements that mark the conclusion of a church service: the doxology, the benediction, the recessional. They may vary from denomination to denomination, from class to class, but there is comfort in the regularity. Each element helps students move mindfully from the mat back into the world, underlining the connection of breath, body, and mind we develop in practice.

From the time you begin to talk students out of savasana, provide them with an orderly sequence of events. This sequence should be one that makes sense to you and that you repeat every time you teach. When it is repeated in class after class, it becomes very soothing for the students.

Revisit the Theme

If you included a theme in class, invite an open-ended exploration of how it's landed. This could be a physical or an emotional cue, and it can be as simple as, "We did lots of hip work tonight; take a few breaths to observe the sensation in your hips," or "We practiced letting go; take a few breaths to continue letting go of what you can."

Align with Intention

Invite students to remember the intention they set at the beginning of practice. Give them time to recommit to that original intention or to rephrase it into a new resolve that works off the mat.

Individual Dedication

After they connect with their own intention, students may like to direct intention outward by offering a dedication of the practice. This could be to a person, an ideal, or to everyone everywhere. It's a nice time for chanting, if that's something you enjoy. A common chant is *Lokah samastah sukhino bhavantu,* May all beings be happy and free. Or simply cue an *om.* Do this explicitly by saying something like, "I invite you to join me in chanting three rounds of *om,* or you may simply listen. We start with a big breath in. *Om, om, om.*" Or: "Join in or listen as we create a sea of *om*s. Join at your pace and in your own key; it will reach a natural conclusion after a few rounds."

Collective Dedication

Finally, move on to collective dedication. We seal this as we recognize each other with *namaste.* If your class is comfortable with it, encourage students to look at each other as they say *namaste.* I cue: "With your next inhalation, lift your gaze, and we'll offer collective dedication with *namaste. Namaste!*" Then I make eye contact with as many students as I can, without unnecessarily prolonging the end.

Call to Action

The end of class is not the time for a lengthy sales pitch, but an until-we-meet-again farewell makes sense. In person, try something like, "I'll see you next week—bring a friend!" or "We'll be investigating these themes all month, hope to see you again," or "If you liked that approach to [any pose, meditation, or theme], I'll be offering a similar workshop...." Finish with a thank-you and move to the door to say goodbye or answer quick questions as students leave.

Make a special point of catching new students, asking how they feel, and calling them by name: "Feel good, George?" If they relaxed deeply, they may not have much to say, so don't take that personally. Even a "yep" can be met with a "Great! I hope to see you next week."

At the end of a video class, make a quick suggestion for next steps, such as: "If you enjoyed this practice, be sure to check out X, Y, and Z, as well as the balance pose tutorial. And sign up for my newsletter at the link on the screen to hear when new videos are posted!" Or, "I'd love to see photos of you practicing this version of tree pose we worked toward. Tag me: @sagerountree!"

Offering a consistent closing is just as important at making students feel welcome as opening class well. As you develop your skill, you'll strengthen both ends of the container to build a strong space for student transformation.

END ON TIME

To lightly paraphrase the words of Judith Lasater, "We start class on time to honor the teacher, we end class on time to honor the students." There is truly no excuse—barring, perhaps, the batteries in the wall clock dying during savasana—for running over your allotted end time. It's unfair to students, who have places to be after class, some of them involving picking up children or catching a bus or moving a car before the parking meter expires. It's unfair to everyone, teacher and students alike, in the class that comes after yours. And it's unfair to the studio itself, as sloppy teachers hurt the studio brand by sending the message, "We're unreliable, and your time doesn't matter to us."

Happily, ending on time or one minute early isn't hard. Do the simple math: Know what time your class needs to end, and work backward from there. How long does it take to guide students gently from savasana through your closing? How many minutes of savasana do you want to offer based on the practice, your students, and the time of day and year, given the 1:10 guideline I mentioned above? Add those together, build in one or two minutes of cushion time, and start savasana with more than enough time to end by or before the official time.

No one has ever complained to me, either as a teacher or as a studio owner, that class ended on time. And no one has ever asked for a prorated discount because class ended one minute early. Not once!

LEAVE THEM WITH SOMETHING SWEET

A really good party might end with a party favor, or the hostess sending home an extra serving of dessert. Perhaps you have something sweet to hand to your students, like a small card with the quote you read in class, or a link to your playlist when students sign up for your newsletter. If so, these can be distributed quietly by each mat during savasana, or you can move to the door to hand them out.

There is typically an awkward moment for the teacher after saying *namaste*. It's far less awkward for students, who are just coming around. Don't immediately jump up and move to the door; move slowly. I usually say, "I'll turn the lights up so you can see your shoes," then I move toward the door.

When you can, stand by the door (but don't block it!), thanking students with eye contact and a smile. "See you next week!" "Hope that felt good." "Thanks for being here." If an individual student has questions for you, angle your body so that you can still glance at people as they are leaving and wave goodbye. If students typically monopolize your time, manage their expectations up front, with something like, "I have five minutes for questions before I have to head to my next appointment." This reinforces healthy boundaries, too, which we will discuss in chapter 9.

9

The Student-Teacher Relationship

· ·

WITHOUT STUDENTS, you wouldn't be a teacher. Your relationship with the people who take your class is precious, and it's critical to your ability to help them with yoga. I'd bet the reason you want to teach is precisely because one or more teachers had a direct positive effect on your life. Excellent! Now you have the chance to pay it forward. Just as your success depends on having a clear vision for your class, your weekly schedule, and your career, so does it depend on taking some time to pinpoint exactly the kind of relationship you want to have with your students. The exercises in this chapter will help.

MAKE YOUR STUDENTS FEEL WELCOME:
CREATING AN INCLUSIVE CLASSROOM

As you develop your class, seek to promote an accepting, inclusive classroom where everyone feels safe and welcome. A good place to start is to avoid talking about burning calories or making up for indiscretions by sweating them out. At the same time, encourage your students to know that their bodies are capable and resilient. Instead of telling students to execute a pose in a particular way to avoid injury, you can say instead that it's often done this way for comfort, or ease, or to fine-tune the amount of stress that goes into a joint. (Stress is not the enemy; excessive stress is.) Keep your language positive.

Be careful to notice if you are assigning value to achieving a certain outcome. For example, do you say, "The ultimate expression of the pose is . . ." If so, why? There are myriad reasons why someone wouldn't be able to take a particular option in any given pose. Some of these are structural, related to the proportion of their bones or the operation of their unique joints—and these will never change. Some are functional, meaning the body hasn't been asked to take a certain movement or hasn't been conditioned to do a particular action. These can change in time, but just because they can, should they?

I recognize that certain styles of yoga subscribe to the idea that there is one "right" way to perform a pose, and that approach filters through the classroom. If you teach in one of these styles, you can explain to your students why things are done in a particular way.

When offering options to students, listen carefully to your language. Weight-lifting coaches might talk about progressions and regressions of an exercise, whereas in yoga we sometimes hear "beginner" or "advanced." But these presume that the "deeper" expression of a pose is more advanced; that's not necessarily true. Instead of "harder" or "easier," I use the terms "spicier" and "sweeter," thinking that casting choices in terms of an individual palate is kinder and allows each student to determine what suits their tastes from one moment to the next.

To keep your classroom inclusive, you should also consider a variety of bodies and learning styles. The length of someone's arm bones relative to their torso can dictate whether they can "successfully" execute a movement without props. Think of staff pose: Some bodies with long torsos can sit in this L shape with arms reaching down and not have palms on the floor; others with long arms can press their palms into the floor and float their seats off the mat. This isn't something that will change with practice; it is what it is. If it suits your class (and staff pose is a pretty good opportunity to do this), take a moment to compare bodies to find the outliers, then show ways to add props so that each student can feel what you are teaching, regardless of body proportion. Making a lesson of these structural differences will free students to meet their bodies where and as they are.

Some students learn by hearing. They will listen to your words and know what to do. Some learn by watching, and they will need to see a demonstration to understand what you are suggesting. Some learn by moving; for these students, practice and manual assists—with consent—will work best. Be sure your class accommodates all learning styles so that every student can understand and participate.

MANAGING STUDENT BEHAVIOR IN CLASS

The vast majority of your students will be wonderful in class. They come to yoga to turn inward, and once they understand the studio etiquette and value the practice, they are dream students. You teach people how to treat you. Once you have established clear boundaries and expectations, 95 percent of your interactions with students will be a joy.

But problems do arise. Below, we will think through how to deal with these common situations. When you find students creating trouble in class, don't be shy in asking for help, even if you feel confident that you can handle the situation on your own. Any issue you've encountered has likely already been addressed at your gym or studio—and sadly, often the problem has already been mentioned to the offending student. Ask the manager or owner for advice and support on how to handle this. Ask your colleagues, too, but be discreet: There's no need to name names or shame students. Your peers may have useful strategies and ideas for you. You aren't alone.

Late Arrivals

Often the students who arrive in class late are the ones with special needs: They're new, or stressed from traffic, or just generally not up to speed on how things operate in your classroom. And you're at a disadvantage, because, once class begins, you're unable to have a regular conversation with them.

When possible, get help from the desk clerk or management. They may hold late arrivals until the class has chanted *om* or begun to move. If you don't have someone to serve as a gatekeeper, signage can be good: "Late arrivals, please enter quietly," or "Late arrivals, please do not enter until the class has begun to move." (Or work around the issue with "This door is locked once class is in session, to protect its integrity. See you next time!") As you fill the room, it's smart to leave space by the door for late arrivals. If needed, you can give them some hand signals to let them know what to do—wave and smile and point to a free spot for them to set up, or raise a finger to indicate they should stand by the door while you mouth "Wait one minute!"

Students Who Would Be Best Served Elsewhere

The number one reason students sign up for a class is schedule: The class is at a time when they can make it. That sometimes means students are in a class that doesn't match their energy level or experience. You'll often have students in class who would do better in a different class—newbies who should check out gentle yoga or a basics series before coming to your dynamic flow class, show-offs (gotta call them what they are!) who are going off-book and distracting your students who came for a mellow class. It's a kindness both to them and to your other students if you can find a gentle way to suggest they try out another class. You might spin this in a flattering way: "Your practice is beautiful! I think you'll love X class with Y teacher on Z-day mornings. I worry that this class wasn't the best use of your time, and I'm really grateful you came." Some of these will self-select. Others will keep coming, at which point you'll need to do a case-by-case assessment of whether to keep them or to express yourself more strongly.

Students Talking/Adjusting Each Other

Students who know each other—parents and children, best friends, romantic partners—can find it tough to focus on their own practice when they are side by side. This is especially true when one of the pair loves yoga and is trying to convince the other how great it is. You might find a student cuing another, or even offering adjustments. When you do, read the situation with empathy, then determine whether to intervene.

If you do think doing something is in order, it can be to lavish extra attention on the newer student (perhaps with a "I've got this; you can focus on your own practice" to the more experienced student). If the vibe in the class is casual enough, you can ask, "Do I need to separate you two?" If all else fails, use the polite yoga code for "Shush it!": "Close your mouth and breathe through your nose."

Students Distracting the Room

Student distractions come in several forms. Students generally distract other students in the room by aggravating the senses of smell, sound, and sight. If a student offends someone else's sense of touch, they should be booted from the room, and let's all hope no one is tasting anyone else in the room!

Smells. Strong smells usually fall into one of these three categories: perfume, smoke, and body odor. Perfume is the simplest to handle. You can make an announcement that since yoga involves deep breathing and people have scent sensitivities, it's common practice to come to class fragrance-free. If someone comes in smelling like they just passed by the department store fragrance counters, you can encourage them to use a wet towel to sponge off what they can.

Smoke is more insidious; it lingers in clothing and in hair. This is a tough one, as developing a regular mindfulness and movement practice can help smokers on the path to quitting. If someone smells strongly of smoke, it's worth reaching out to say, "I notice you might live with a smoker. Can you help me think of ways to reduce the smell for the benefit of the whole class? Would it be helpful to store a set of yoga clothes in your car or at the studio for you to change into?" Asking the student to help come up with a solution can keep them feeling included and involved instead of excluded and judged.

Toughest of all is the student with strong body odor. There are many permutations of this issue, from the student who comes in clean but develops a strong smell when the class heats up, to a student who seems to willfully disregard societal norms of hygiene. In the former case, there may not be much to be done; in the latter, you'll need to have a discussion. Again, ask the student to help you find a solution.

Sounds. Deep breathing can be loud, and a gentle sigh sometimes morphs into an ecstatic moan. Some classes and studios actively promote this; others don't! Know the culture where you're teaching, so that you can understand what students expect a class to sound like. If you have a single student repeatedly moaning and groaning, it might be time to say, "Let's get out all our sounds with a few rounds of lion's breath," or "This should feel good, it shouldn't hurt."

If a student begins snoring during savasana, quietly move over to them and gently squeeze their ankles. That's usually enough to pull them out of sleep. Sometimes they will even stop upon your approach.

If you are teaching a live-streaming class, it generally makes sense to mute all students as you begin. Be sure that, as the host/organizer, you know how to use the software to mute, if someone—or their pet or child—starts to make distracting noises.

Sights. Students are in class for their own practice, and modifications are critical to each student's receiving what they need from your class. But someone going completely rogue may distract the whole class and can even be dangerous. (Have you been in a class where a renegade handstander randomly started kicking up in the middle of the room? I have; it is not a relaxing experience for the students!) You'll need to decide where to draw the line between letting such a student have their own experience and letting them derail the class.

This is likely a game-time decision. Some people just want attention! Others have valid reasons for their modifications. Lately, I've said, "You're free to go off-book as long as you don't interfere with your neighbors."

Combos. Students entering late or leaving class early combine distracting sounds and sights. Recognizing that the culture in some regions and styles is that savasana is optional and left to the student's discretion, I suggest you emphasize the importance of savasana if you expect students to stay for the entire period. When you know a student has to leave early, suggest they depart before savasana begins. Be sure to manage student expectations around savasana by mentioning how long it will last, why we do it, what to do if it's not relaxing, and when the class will be moving out. These set up a condition where students can best enjoy their relaxation, and once they enjoy it, they will be less likely to leave.

All this advice boils down to: "Build a strong container." Let your students know with your words and your actions what is acceptable. Once you've set this expectation, manage it consistently and kindly. The great majority of your students will learn quickly and become models for the rest of the class.

Practice Your Approach

Draft three approaches, with the language you'd want to use, to these issues. What would you say, when and how?

▶ A student carries a very strong odor

▶ A student leaves loudly during savasana

▶ A student goes way off-book during class, and students appear to be distracted

Communication: In Person, Phone, or Email?

Sensitive conversations are difficult. Just thinking about bringing up someone's body odor may cause *you* to break out in a sweat. Use your judgment about your student and your own communication skills to discern the most compassionate way to have these conversations. If a student is prone to aggression, email or phone may be best. Sending a written message gives the student time to process it in their own way, and space to compose a level response. That said, don't choose email simply because it's the least confrontational option—a friendly smile and even some visible discomfort can soften the blow of hearing that your body odor is affecting the class, and in that case a face-to-face conversation may be the kindest choice.

Electronic Devices

With the ubiquity of smartphones and smart watches, students are accustomed to having screens at hand every moment. A yoga class offers a chance to turn away from the constant barrage of incoming messages and toward inner experience. Having screens in class interferes with this opportunity, so whenever possible, encourage your students leave their phones in their cars or bags, and that they put their smart watches on Do Not Disturb as well as Theater Mode so that they are not distracted by incoming messages, and their neighbors are not distracted by their screen lighting up. Even cell phones set to vibrate can make an ungodly racket, especially if they are resting directly on a wooden table or bench.

There are valid reasons for a student to have a phone in class: They may be a medical professional or emergency services worker on call, or attending their first yoga class while leaving a new baby with a caregiver. If possible, encourage these students to leave their devices with the staff covering the front desk; they will be able to relax better and the desk staff can get them if needed. If it's necessary, set these students up toward the back of the room with the phone shielded from students' view. Any other use of a phone in class can be discouraged with a simple reminder like, "This is your time to connect your body, mind, and breath—and your phone is not invited to this party." If you are using a wireless microphone to record video in class, the signal from cell phones can interfere. Ask students to turn their phones off or to put them in airplane mode.

Of course, the same rule that applies to your students goes for you! It is highly unprofessional for a teacher to be touching a phone during class for any reason other than a quick volume or soundtrack change in class. Do not answer texts while your students are in savasana. Do not, under any circumstances, take unannounced photos of your students without their explicit consent, especially during savasana. If you use a smart watch, which can be a great device for timing longer holds of poses and for controlling your music, mention to your students what you are doing ("I'm setting a timer as we take a yin yoga–style hold of this pose"). Be sure your own device is in Do Not Disturb and your watch is in Theater Mode.

Unless a student is answering phone calls in the room, stick to blanket announcements directed to the whole room and save any individual conversations for after class. You never know exactly what's happening. I once saw a student fiddling with what I presumed was her pager throughout a workshop I taught. The session was almost over when I realized it was a blood sugar monitor!

Script It

Draft a few different ways to express quickly to students that phones are not welcome in class.

Family Members in Class

At the start of your teaching career, your students may be primarily people you know and have invited to class. You may even have created a class for your friends and family to gain experience. Great! However: Make it clear how long this situation will be in effect. If you are teaching your friends for free, how long will you do it? Four weeks? Two months? Have an answer other than "indefinitely."

The toughest student for me to have in class is my husband, Wes. He's used to having my attention in a very specific way, and my attention goes right to him even in a room full of students. The lines of communication between us were laid down in 1995, and they are very different from how I communicate with my other students. You might find something similar happening in your class.

Conversely, our daughter Lillian is my best source of constructive feedback about my teaching. She can pinpoint my filler phrases and overused words, and, as a teenager, can spot anything phony in my affect in front of the class. As a studio owner, I find it difficult to get an honest critique even from other teachers (I hired them, so I get it), and Lillian's advice is invaluable.

When you have family members in class, let your students know who they are. Not only do students like a peek into your personal life—and it's just a peek—such introductions also explain any intimacy evident between you and your family, so they help manage student expectations of the appropriate teacher-student rapport.

INJURIES AND SCOPE OF PRACTICE

While it seems counterintuitive, I suggest you do *not* ask students about their injuries. Legally, once you are aware of these injuries, you are responsible for them. And realistically, what are you going to do with a room full of various complaints? Instead, encourage each student to take responsibility for their personal health. Cut out the extra time and jump right to that step. Remind students early and often that everything is optional, nothing should hurt, and that it's always OK to move out of something that doesn't feel right in favor of rest. Mention common modifications, like having hands to your heart or your hips if lifting your arms overhead doesn't feel good for your shoulders.

Students may announce an injury to you uninvited; don't freak out if they do. Ask the student if they have been cleared by their medical providers to do the physical movements of class. It would be within your rights to refuse to have a student in class without a note from their health-care team.

Know your scope of practice. If you are a physical therapist, you should be paid a physical therapist's rates in your clinic to answer students' questions—that's outside the purview of yoga. Don't hesitate to say, "That's outside my knowledge base," or, if you do have a practice that covers the issue, "That's beyond the bounds of this class, but it is something I can address in an appointment at my office. Here's how to book one."

Develop a network of providers you can refer students to. This could include a sports medicine clinic, an orthopedist, a chiropractor, a massage therapist, and so on. If you're not sure which providers would be a good choice, ask at your local running store. They likely have a network of clinicians who are used to working with people with movement-related injuries.

Handling Different Bodies and Special Needs

A healthy attachment to exercise and to the benefits of yoga is a good thing. Too much of that good thing can lead to overdoing it, a condition called *orthorexia*. If you have a student in many classes in a day, it's fine to make a general comment like, "You've really gone all in on your practice!" But listen carefully to the student's answers. As a teacher, you are not in a position to diagnose students, or to tell them exactly how much is too much. But you can talk about the importance of rest, and the law of diminishing returns, in which some exercise is great but too much doesn't yield better results. When in doubt, talk to your studio owner and yoga mentors rather than directly approaching a student.

If you teach an open class, you are likely to have pregnant students. Sometimes you won't know they are pregnant—sometimes *they* won't know yet that they are pregnant! Being conversant in how to adapt for each of the trimesters will make this a smoother experience for both you and your student once the pregnancy is public. Linda Sparrowe's *Yoga Mama: The Practitioner's Guide to Prenatal Yoga* will help.

   In both these cases, be careful not to reach a conclusion based on how a body presents in class. Someone who looks pregnant to you might not be! Worse, they might be trying hard to conceive, have just lost a pregnancy, or recently given birth, and your words can hurt. Similarly, don't equate a slim body with exercise addiction. Bodies come in various shapes and sizes, and we all benefit when no one judges the book by its cover.

IN CASE OF EMERGENCY

The more you teach, the greater the probability of something going wrong in your class, from heart attacks to fart attacks. Thinking through how you might handle such emergencies will make them easier to handle in the moment. Be sure you have covered these bases.

Logistics

Know where you are. What is the physical location of your classroom? How will you direct emergency services to find you if you need an ambulance or firefighters?

Know where the closest AED is. An AED—automated external defibrillator—can help reset heart rhythms and is an important resource in the case of a cardiac event. If your class is in a gym or in a studio in a shopping center, there may be an AED nearby. Scope it out, and consider how you could direct a student to find it in case of an emergency. ("Jeff, run to Kroger's across the parking lot for the AED!")

Know the number for emergency services. If you are teaching internationally, be aware of how to to reach emergency services wherever you are. Students will help you with this.

Know CPR and first aid. If you haven't taken a CPR class in the last two years, look for one offered by the Red Cross, the American Heart Association, or a similar organization. Even refreshing your memory in an online course is better than not knowing anything. Some gyms and studios will require you maintain CPR certification, and some of these pay to provide it for you. And fear not: If you need to call emergency services and CPR is warranted, they will talk you through what to do. It's also a good idea to learn how to use an EpiPen on someone suffering a severe allergic reaction—they may carry the pen but be unable to instruct you.

People Management

Keep eyes on your class. If someone looks dizzy or wobbly, discreetly put them in a resting pose like child's pose or legs up the wall, or bring them to sit on a cushion. Check in with students if they leave the room. Be subtle: Don't yell, "Hey, where ya going?" A simple thumbs-up sign or OK sign with raised eyebrows and a slight frown can convey your concern. If someone has been gone for a while, send a regular student (if it's feasible) to check on them. They may be having a GI emergency, or a heart attack—in women, the symptoms can register the same.

Delegate. If someone loses consciousness, delegate. Point to one student and have them call emergency services, then send another out to meet the ambulance. Ask if anyone in the class has medical training. If so, let them take charge; your role becomes keeping your students calm. If the emergency warrants, send students home. Sometimes loss of consciousness or seizures are accompanied by a loss of bowel control, or vomiting. If that happens, obviously class will not continue, and it's better to clear the room of all nonessential people.

Emergency contact. Many enrollment software programs require that students enter an emergency contact. If you have desk staff, ask them to contact this individual; if not, do this yourself as soon as is feasible. You might also find an emergency contact in the sick student's phone. On most smartphones, you can activate the screen, then choose "Emergency." Emergency contacts may be entered under that name—"emergency contact"—or as ICE ("in case of emergency").

Document. Once the situation is resolved and you have taken a few deep breaths, send an email to your manager explaining what happened and the steps you took. This should happen in any emergency involving bodily fluids or loss of consciousness—even if it's just a student cutting herself on a nail that's popped up from the floor. If your class is at a gym or a similarly large organization, they may have an incident report form for you to complete. Even if you're teaching a class that you're hosting on your own, or a private lesson, document what happened and save it. This may be important down the road. If you needed to dismiss the class and *only if you have the sick student's express permission*, you can follow up with students to say how everything was resolved.

When the Emergency Is Yours

Sometimes the emergency is your own: You are suddenly stricken midclass with acute nausea, bowel pain, a coughing fit, or a migraine. In such cases, simply do your best. If you become ill during class, use your best judgment about what to do. (I have a colleague who once put students into a pose, ran from the room with morning sickness, then returned to continue on the second side.) If there is an experienced teacher or student in the room, deputize them to hold the space while you care for yourself. If there is a front desk, alert them to what's up. It is OK for you to cancel class or end early if you are suddenly unwell, especially if you realize you are coming down with something that might be contagious. No matter how much your students appreciate how they feel after taking your class, none of them are in such dire need of yoga that they couldn't join the next class or next week's class.

Planning Is Indispensable

Imagine a scenario in which you suddenly feel sick during class. How will you handle this? Write it out as one or more if/then statements. You may never need to use these plans, but if you do, having run them through in your imagination will be useful.

MANAGING YOUR REACTION TO STUDENTS:
DROP THE STORY

You'll never know what your students are thinking. Often it's the student with the most inscrutable expression who is having the deepest experience. Don't fear the resting bitch face! A slightly furrowed brow is often the sign of someone paying attention or concentrating. If you look out and see a room full of smiles and hear laughter at every quip you offer, your students are focusing on you, not the inner experience. At that point, you're entertaining them, not facilitating their experience in self-discovery.

While this is true of all age groups, it's especially the case with tweens and teens. Don't get caught up in trying to elicit smiles; don't tell yourself stories about what the students are thinking. Just teach the yoga as authentically as you can. And be true to yourself: No one can smell a phony like a teenager. Use your own words, your own voice. Don't simply parrot your favorite teacher or put on airs.

I've mentioned to rooms of experienced teachers that I find the students who leave quickest after class often had the deepest experience. They always agree. More than once, I've gotten a note from the students with the most unreadable faces saying, "That was just what I needed today." Here are a few stories that underscore how we can never know what people are thinking from their expressions.

First, I was leading a teachers' intensive in a room with poor acoustics and I encouraged students to draw close to me so I wouldn't have to yell to be heard. While many moved their mats, one remained outside the semicircle. I asked her by name to come near us, and she scooted forward on her mat only a foot or so. Figuring it was a lost cause, I continued and hoped she could hear me. At the end of the five-day workshop, she told me, "I know you wanted me to come closer that first day. But I'd just been in the hospital with my son, who had the flu, and the doctor said I might be contagious for 24 hours. I really wanted to be in the workshop, but I didn't want to infect anyone—that's why I did what I did."

My colleague Alexandra was once teaching when a student packed up and left in the middle of class, gesturing that she was sorry. Alexandra had once taught a class where a woman had a stroke (happily, the student's husband was with her, whisked her off to the hospital, and she recovered), so she worried that that this student may have been sick. After class, Alexandra sat down to send her a message. While she did, an email came in from the student. She'd had a creeping feeling that she left the kettle on the stove with the burner on, she said, and when she got home, she found it dry and glowing red.

To add one more story, this one from outside yoga: I was heading to my regular step aerobics class (this was 1996, the heyday of step) when my father called to tell me my grandmother had died. After hanging up, I continued what I was doing on autopilot and went to the gym. Only 15 minutes into the routine did it strike me: I did *not* want to be at step aerobics! I packed up my equipment and left, explaining it to the teacher at the next class. My leaving had absolutely zero to do with her.

Finally, even though you're striving to be a kind, accepting person, do you like every single being you come into contact with? Of course not. Sometimes the vibe just isn't right. The same thing will go for your students. Don't hold them to a standard you wouldn't hold yourself to.

MANAGING STUDENT BEHAVIOR OUTSIDE OF CLASS: SETTING BOUNDARIES

What happens in class will inform your relationship with your students outside of class. When you have clear boundaries in the classroom, students are likely to respect your personal space and your time outside the classroom. But the very thing that makes students feel great in class—seeing you, their teacher, as a sympathetic caretaker—can lead students to assign you as the cause. While this is a natural projection, remind students that you are not the source of their positive feelings—their own yoga practice is. Issue this reminder whenever you find that students are deifying you. This might come in the form of compliments after class, or in a request for more guidance or attention (an invitation to coffee, for example). The higher the pedestal your students put you on, the more painful it will be for them when they realize you're a typical messy human. Don't lay your dark secrets bare to them, but do remind them that you are just a person with flaws and that their positive reaction to yoga is due not to you but to their own good work on the mat.

The gold standard on the ethics around teacher-student relationships is laid out in black-and-white terms in Donna Farhi's book *Teaching Yoga: Exploring the Teacher-Student Relationship.* This book is well worth your time. In your day-to-day life, you'll find there are far more gray areas. The modern studio generally doesn't elevate teachers to guru status (with some notable exceptions), so the power dynamic is often not as strong as you'll see it described in Farhi's book or other accounts of appropriate ethics. If you choose to register with the Yoga Alliance, you'll sign their general Code of Conduct. It binds you to maintaining standards of professionalism—ensuring student safety, creating an inclusive classroom, appropriately setting and fulfilling expectations.

Below are common situations you may encounter and suggestions on how to handle them professionally. In each of these, you should be polite and kind without inviting further complication. Putting a little space between you and the student—saying, "Sorry, I need to leave for my next class," for example—will give you some time to contemplate an efficient and appropriate answer, and to consult with your manager and your mentor before proceeding.

How to Communicate

In general, your communication with students will take place either in person within the studio or in the context of one-to-many marketing, which we discussed above. If students reach out to you by direct message on your social media or by asking for your phone number, please know that you do not need to answer any message or to share your contact information. You can direct any inquiry to your studio owner, or you may simply ignore it.

If you are teaching online, students may comment on your videos, depending on the platform. If you have the energy, you can respond to each comment with a quick "thank you." Recognize that you'll be setting a precedent! While responding to comments can be a great way to build an audience, it can also become a drain on your time.

You may need to text your students to confirm a private appointment. Be sure to keep these communications professional—treat texts as though they were emails. Use proper punctuation and be brief and clear.

What to Communicate

If a student asks you for advice on choosing a class, retreat, or teacher training, be honest but professional. Don't engage in gossip about other students or teachers. A good rule of thumb: Don't say anything you wouldn't broadcast to your entire newsletter list or want your grandmother to hear.

Personal Friendships

Some of your students may come in as preexisting friends of yours. Others might be the kind of person you would like to have as a friend. Being friendly with your students is different from being their friend. Don't issue an invitation to one student that you would not give the entire class. If a group of students invites you out socially after class, either politely decline or be sure the invitation has been clearly issued to the entire class.

Romantic Relationships

Never capitalize on your status as teacher to leverage relationships with your students. This is a clear, unethical abuse of power. If a potential for a romantic relationship emerges, talk to your supervisor and your mentors. So much depends on the power dynamic at play. For example, a teacher trainer clearly should never date a trainee during or immediately after the course of the program. But what about going on a date with someone who once accompanied a friend to your class—maybe exactly because that friend thought you two would get along? What about inviting a new romantic interest to your class? When can your partner begin attending your class? Once you live together? Once you are married? These are situations with less clear-cut parameters. The grayer the situation, the more important it is that you talk to your mentorship team about what to do. Take your time. Any relationship worth waiting for can stand a slow unfolding. If you're feeling rushed or under pressure, that's a good sign that you should *not* pursue a relationship. Remember the *yama* of *brahmacharya*. It's sometimes translated as "sexual chastity." I prefer the interpretation of *brahmacharya* as temperance: deliberate self-control.

Gifts

Receiving gifts from students should be considered on an ad-hoc basis and with awareness of your workplace's stated policy. (If one isn't stated, ask.) It would be rude to turn down, say, a dozen eggs from your student's chicken coop or a book that your student thinks you will enjoy, but it might make sense to turn down invitations to drinks or gifts of clothing or jewelry. Whenever possible, keep the gift at the studio rather than taking it home. It removes some of the potential pitfalls of a personal gift-giving relationship while sharing the sentiment with the entire studio community. We sometimes have students bring us flowers, which stay at the studio for everyone to enjoy, or little statues from their trips that can go on a windowsill or altar.

Draft Your Response

Since you may be tongue-tied when a student approaches you with a gift or a request for a date, it's useful in advance to think through some polite ways to turn the student down. Draft a response to these prompts. Think of how you can deflect and redirect the attention.

"Can I take you out for coffee? I have some questions about yoga."

"Can I take you out for coffee? I'd like to get to know you better."

"Will you tell me about XYZ studio? I'm considering doing their teacher training and wondered if it's the right fit for me."

"Will you tell me about XYZ studio? I heard some freaky cult stuff goes down over there."

"Your class has made me feel so good, I'd like to repay you with this gift certificate for a massage."

"Your class has made me feel so good, I'd like to repay you by giving you a massage myself."

It's good to have thought through these potential pitfalls so that you'll be less surprised if you encounter them. But virtually all of your work with students will be positive and satisfying. These positive relationships are a form of yoga—connection. In part 4, we'll look at ways you can connect beyond the regular class.

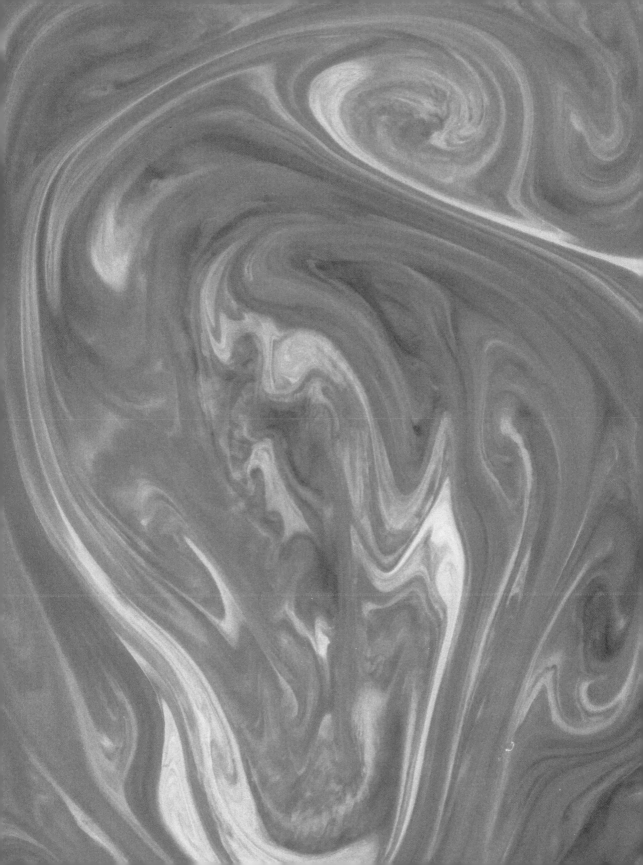

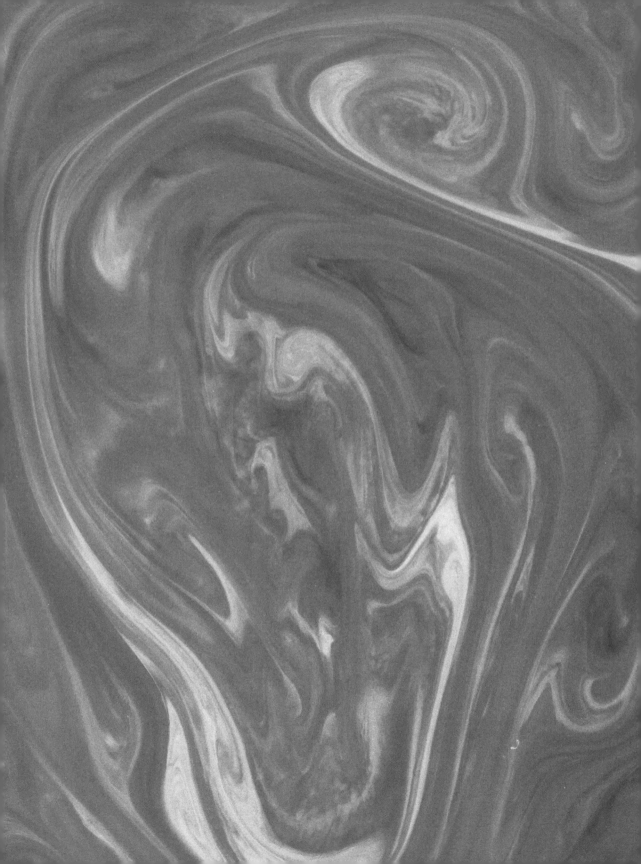

PART 4

Leveling Up as a Teacher

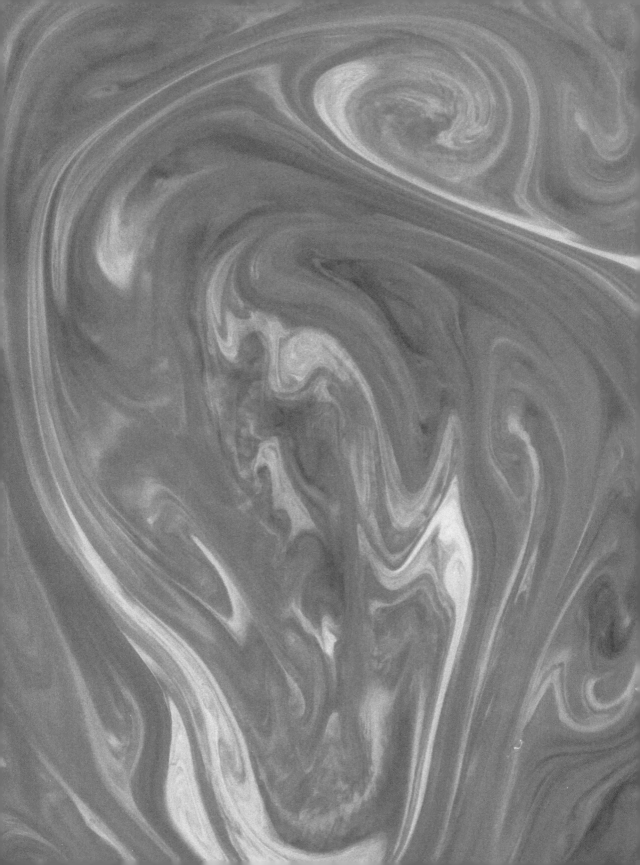

10
Beyond the Regular Class

· ·

WHILE TEACHING A WEEKLY CLASS at a gym or a studio is likely to be your first gig as a yoga teacher, there are many other opportunities for you to teach. Outside of the gym or studio, you might set up your own one-person shop offering regular or occasional sessions at a community center, house of worship, art gallery, or park. And beyond the weekly class format, you might offer one-time workshops, limited-run series, retreats, private lessons, fundraiser classes, and online content. Let's explore locations and platforms for these teaching options and the best way to plan, execute, and evaluate them professionally.

DIY: THE ONE-PERSON PHYSICAL STUDIO

Find a Location

Cast a wide net to find a good location to host your in-person classes. Think of spaces that have downtime at the times you'd like to teach. This could include school gymnasiums, houses of worship or community centers, dance studios, or parks. Give deep consideration to parking availability and accessibility via public transit, depending on typical methods of transportation in your area. You want it to be as easy as possible for people to get to your class.

If you are going to teach on your own, you'll need a space that has room for enough mats for you to pass breaking even and earn money. A yoga mat is generally 2 feet (0.5 m) wide and 5½ feet (2 m) long, so you'll want a space of at least 4 feet (1 m) by 7 feet (2 m), or 28 square feet (2.5 m²), for each student, plus cushioning around the sides of the room and space for you. (If you are in a dense metropolitan area, you may go tighter, as your students may be accustomed to having less space between mats and generally used to sharing tighter quarters with other humans.) I suggest giving more space per student: 40 to 50 square feet (4–5 m²) per person.

You'll likely pay a flat fee per hour to rent the space. Be sure you are clear on when you are allowed to come, whether and how you are expected to clean, and the length of your contract. Get this in writing, and run it past an attorney to be extra clear. As you secure your rental, you need to be sure you're going to clear enough students in class to cover the fee and to earn you a profit. Consider whether and how you can cancel the contract if you aren't getting traction.

If you are teaching outside on public property, like a municipal park, you will likely need a permit from the town. Be careful to research and secure what you need long before you plan to start teaching, as permits can get tied up in bureaucracy. Obviously, if you are outside, you'll need an inclement-weather plan and clear communication with your students about how and when any cancellations or rain locations will be conveyed: on your website, social media, email list or newsletter, or all of the above.

Be sure your liability coverage extends to any physical location you rent, and check that the venue also has its own insurance covering the building itself (entry and exit).

Finally, consider equipment. Are you going to buy enough mats, blocks, blankets, and other props to outfit your entire class? If so, where will you store them and how will you transport them into and out of class? Are you asking students to bring their own materials? If so, you might be able to sell them props to enhance your bottom line. Students would buy from you, then carry their own props to and from class.

Promote

Decide who your student base will be—this may depend on the location of the space you're renting, and it may target the people who already visit the space. Then figure out where they are spending time, so you can decide how best to market your classes to them. For example, if you are teaching yoga at a boathouse in a vacation town, you can post flyers at the venue and in other places vacationers visit during the week: the rental agency, the local grocery store, the ice cream shop, and so on.

If you expect students to bring their own props, make this clear in your promotion. This could be as simple as "bring a beach towel and sunscreen" for outdoor classes.

Set Pricing and Payment

Figure out a pay structure that makes sense. Say you are teaching on a beach—and of course, you have taken care to get the town's permission. Do you expect an audience of locals, or of weekenders and/or vacationers? If the former, you might offer a low rate for a series to folks who can show proof of residency; for the latter, single drop-ins at a higher price make sense. Or perhaps you'll offer both to incentivize a broader range of students to come to class.

Decide how to take payment. Do you want students to pay only in advance online so that you don't need to handle class fees immediately before and after you teach? Or do you find it easy enough to process cards using an app like Square or Stripe on your phone? If you are selling a class pass, devise an easy way to keep track of how many classes students have left. This could be a spreadsheet, a paper notebook that you photograph weekly in case of loss (store the photos in the cloud), or an online scheduling or event software.

DIY: THE ONE-PERSON VIRTUAL STUDIO

Find a Location

Even when you're teaching virtually, you still need a home for your classes. This could be directly on your website, using uploaded or embedded videos, or via a plug-in housed on your website. In the former scenario, you'd upload videos to your site, YouTube, or Vimeo, and set the videos to private mode or protect them with a password, then sell access to your viewers. This is a way to test the waters or get started sharing free content to build your brand.

The next level would be using a video-on-demand platform to handle delivery and sales, freeing you from having to manage viewers' access to videos. These platforms handle payment, and they generally allow you to customize the presentation of videos, so you have a consistent brand identity between the main page and the video platform. These include Namastream, Pivotshare, and Vimeo Pro. Visit yogateacherhandbook. com for a list of platforms to consider.

Promote

Promoting your online studio starts with generating some short, helpful video clips that demonstrate what you have to offer. Record and edit several of these, keeping them under three minutes long. Try to teach something in each one: a fun use for a prop, a mantra, a breath technique. These could even be snippets from your longer video. Include a call to action: "Find more tips like this at my online studio!" "Sign up for my newsletter for more of these!" Add captions for accessibility and viewers' ease of use. Then, share the clips liberally.

As part of this sharing, you might boost a social media post or make an advertisement out of your video. Depending on who your target audience is, you can really dial-in your online advertising.

Most important in promoting your offerings online: Be unabashedly yourself! If you're goofy, lean in. If you're strong, highlight that. If you play live music in savasana, show it! First off, it's easier to be who you are, and secondly, it's what will draw your unique audience to you.

Set Pricing and Payment

There are three options for pricing online content: selling a subscription, offering a short-term rental, or making the content available for purchase (either as a download or lifetime access). Some combination of these will likely work for you.

Subscriptions help your bottom line by generating recurring revenue. Once you have a library of several videos, and especially if you are regularly updating your content, subscriptions offer value to the user: They can access whatever they like in any order based on their available time and needs.

Rentals are a good entry point; they let users sample the content without committing much time or money to a purchase or subscription. You may offer a free rental as an incentive for people to sign up for your newsletter, or let your friends share a code for a free rental.

Purchases make sense in some contexts, especially if you are writing in addition to video. E-books and PDFs outlining yoga exercises can be a nice complement to follow-along video content.

A combination of all three may work best, with price points that make it easy for users to choose what's best for them. My Core Strength for Real People series, hosted by Vimeo On Demand but housed at corestrength.sagerountree.com, is priced at $9.99 per month for a subscription, $1.99 per 48-hour rental, or $3.99 per video for purchase. I offer a free rental code for newsletter subscribers, which is included in their welcome email.

If you're using a video-on-demand platform, you may pay a monthly fee for the service or share a cut of what your videos earn. Projecting forward several months, to estimate what you might earn, will help you choose between platforms.

Launch with a Catalog and a Plan

As you produce the content for your studio, start by developing a catalog of several videos—both longer follow-along videos and shorter instructional ones. These longer videos may be anywhere from ten to sixty-plus minutes long. If you are offering a subscription library, instead of recording one very long video as though it were an in-person class, consider breaking it into segments: centering, warm-up, movement, stillness, closing. Then, students can link these segments together to choose their own adventure—à la carte, as it were. You can also offer a full, fixed menu of a long practice as a stand-alone purchase.

The shorter instructional videos can be demonstrations of prop usage, alignment or action in a pose, or anything that would be useful for the viewer to learn outside of the context of a follow-along video. These include short videos where you introduce yourself, tell relevant stories about how you learned to do a certain pose, or share how you overcame an obstacle using yoga. Students will enjoy knowing about you and your background—and the more you show your personality while staying professional, the more loyal your customer base will be.

As you work on these videos, you will edit them a little or a lot. Editing can be as simple as using your photo-editing software to trim off the excess video at the start and end of your class—or as sophisticated as using video-editing software to add transitions, B-roll, voice-over, or other effects. If you misspoke, forgot a pose and started a sequence over to include it, or otherwise flubbed something, you can edit it out at this stage. If you use a Mac or an iOS device, iMovie is a good starter editor, as is Lightworks or Kapwing on a Windows system or any browser, and Adobe Premiere Clip on Android. If you are looking for a full-featured program, Adobe Premiere Pro and Final Cut Pro will offer additional options, though they are far more complex than you need to start. At the very least, prepare a title card: a graphic introducing your content. This can be still or animated, and it will include the title of the series, possibly the episode title, and your name. At the end of the video, insert any credits and a graphic pointing viewers to your website or suggesting some other action to take.

Be sure to amass a decent library—at least five longer videos and five to ten shorter videos—before launching the platform. That way, it will immediately demonstrate its value to people who consider subscribing or buying. It may make sense to have several longer classes available at launch, with several more finished and ready to be uploaded on a regular schedule. This will help retain your initial subscribers.

When you set this schedule, don't be overly ambitious! One or two new videos per month should be plenty. You can always add content more frequently than you planned; but once you have promised to add more on a particular schedule, you're committed to it.

Audio Can Be Lovely

Video is not for everybody. And for some practices, video is irrelevant. If you teach yoga nidra, meditation, or breath work, you may choose to create audio content instead of video. Most of the advice still applies here: launch with several options, house the long-form content behind a paywall, and use short snippets to promote. You may even find that audio-only content adds value: Your users can enjoy your teaching when they're awake in bed at night or traveling on a plane.

Beyond the regular class, whether at a studio, retreat center, or DIY location, you might reach students with a workshop, series, or retreat. Here's how to get started.

DEVELOPING WORKSHOPS

A workshop is generally a onetime event focused on a limited topic that takes place in a day or over a weekend. Think of it like a feature film: It should be able to stand alone, though it might leave room for a sequel. If you can envision more than two meetings for this workshop, you can develop it as a series, which we discuss below. All of the steps you'd take to develop a workshop will apply to series, too. And both workshops and series can be offered as online courses—detailed in what follows. Here is how to create, plan, place, and promote a workshop. (I also cover this topic in the Workshop Workshop at sageyogateachertraining.com.)

Identify and Define Your Topic

You may get an idea for a workshop based on something you see your students working with in class. Maybe you realize they need to learn the basics of chaturanga, or sun salutations. Maybe they want to learn more about pranayama. Workshops can also be keyed to the seasons: You could do a workshop on surrender and letting go for the autumnal equinox, for example, or on setting intentions for New Year's Day. Or you can pitch a workshop to people who participate in an activity: yoga for gardeners, yoga for bridge players, and so on. Or target a life situation: combating infertility, coping with grief, dealing with osteopenia and osteoporosis.

A good workshop has a very clear vision of its topic. To sharpen your understanding, ask yourself the five Ws and one H. Home in on the problem (the what) that your students (the who) will relate to. Ask yourself where and when and why they encounter that problem. Then plan to solve it with yoga—the how.

Focus on Your Topic

Spend some time considering what you have to teach and to whom. Write in response to these prompts:

▶ Who are your students? These can be your current students or the students in a location where you plan to offer a workshop.

- What is a problem your students have? This could be not feeling ready for a handstand, or having back pain after gardening, or feeling anxious before standardized testing.
- When do they encounter this problem?
- Where do they encounter this problem?
- Why does this problem emerge? From your answer here, you'll be able to see the solution.
- How can you use yoga or movement to address this problem?

Write a Description and Title

A good description and title set out the road map for you and your students. It guides your students to see themselves in the workshop, and it sets the agenda that you'll flesh out in your class planning. A good description hits these notes:

- Recognize a problem.
- Propose a solution.
- Explain the methods.
- Project the results.
- Define who this is for (beginners or teachers) and not for (anyone with major injuries, for example).
- Include the price and when and how to register.

Here's the description I wrote when I developed my Workshop Workshop as a three-hour in-person offering:

Are you eager to share your favorite topics with your students in workshop format but unsure about where and how to begin? In this workshop on developing workshops, studio co-owner and yoga teacher training lead teacher Sage Rountree explains the who, what, where, why, when, and how of creating, locating a home for, marketing, and teaching successful workshops—from one-hour sessions to weeklong intensives to retreats to ongoing series.

In lecture, discussion, journaling, and small-group work, you'll identify what you have to offer, refine your vision, write a description that will encourage students to sign up, create a lesson plan and resources to provide students, develop a marketing plan, and workshop the workshop itself with your supportive colleagues.

This workshop is appropriate for teachers of all styles of yoga and movement arts. Bring your tablet, laptop, or notebook, as well as your workshop ideas and questions. You'll leave with a fully developed offering to benefit both your students and your own career.

$75; $65 before 3/1

3 Yoga Alliance continuing education credits

Sign up here [with a link]

Once you've got the description written, you can title your workshop. It could be Yoga for X, where X is the problem you've identified, or Yoga vs. X. Or, if it's an introductory workshop, how about X 101, X Basics, or Fundamentals of X? You can also add a subtitle, something like "The Workshop Workshop: Designing and Leading Transformational Programs," or "Yoga for Athletes: Strength, Flexibility, and Focus." Your title should consider the voice or tone and culture of the host studio. The studio may even have suggestions or input.

Draft a Description and Title

Using the model above, write a description for a workshop designed to help students solve the problem you defined in the previous exercise. Hit these notes:

▶ Define a problem.

▶ Propose a solution.

▶ Explain the methods.

▶ Project the results.

▶ Explain who this is for (beginners or teachers) and not for (anyone with major injuries, for example).

▶ Include the price and when and how to register.

Plan Your Lessons

Working from the expectations you've set in the description, plan what you'll do, why, and how you'll do it, while noting an estimate of how long each portion of the workshop will take. Be sure to balance stillness and movement and, if relevant, personal work like journaling or asana practice with small- and full-group work and discussions. Plan more than you need, and designate which activities could expand, contract, or be cut altogether.

Repetition is the key to learning. Repeat your central message early and often, and be sure all the activities you have planned are tied in to this message.

You'll want your students to have a clear takeaway from the workshop: a sense that they have learned something they can apply in their lives on or off the mat. This could be a handout, a video you send a link to, or something else, like an outline explaining a homework exercise.

Lesson Planning

Using this format or one that makes better sense for your teaching style, write a lesson plan for the workshop. Be sure to consider what could be cut for time; you might choose to highlight it in a different color.

Time in class	What you'll do	Why you'll do it	How you'll do it	How long it will take, with ways to contract or expand

Teach or Record the Workshop

A workshop is, in many ways, a lot like a class, and all my advice about setting up for and leading a class applies. In other ways, workshops are different. They generally last longer than a regular class, so you may want to offer a scheduled comfort break. If you're leading a daylong or weekend workshop, there will be breaks for meals. Be clear with students on how long each break is and when, where, and how you will reconvene—"Let's take fifteen minutes and meet back here at 11:45, sitting in a circle. I'll sound the chime at 11:45."

If you are recording your workshop for delivery online, divide its content into digestible lessons. These videos should last around twenty minutes or less (this makes it easier for your students to process and for file management.) Students can move through the course little by little, at a pace that allows time for them to integrate the lessons. Collect any materials that will complement your lessons: not only your lecture and practice but also slides, illustrations, video clips, and so on. Written material can be offered as downloads, and illustrations and clips can be edited directly into your video. These extra materials make your video far richer and more engaging than a simple, unbroken recording of you talking.

Introduce yourself and your workshop with a clear road map of where you're going and how you'll get there. This reiterates the expectations you set in the title and description, and it establishes a baseline so students can feel that their expectations are met.

In addition to lecture and led practice, some workshops can leave room for full-group or small-group discussion. Inviting a discussion can feel like a pleasant loosening of the reins, but remember that as the leader, you're still the one responsible for keeping class on track. Some students will take advantage of discussion time or Q&A time to tell stories that aren't really questions. To stay on the rails, you may sometimes need to say, "Great question," or "Interesting story, but it's outside the purview of this workshop. Does anyone else have a question on our current topic that it would help everyone to hear answered?" If you are going to leave room for questions, slot this time *before* savasana. After savasana, especially the luxuriously long savasana that workshops afford, students won't feel much like talking—if they even remember their questions.

In the context of a onetime workshop, it's likely unnecessary to do a long period of student introductions. These can take forever and contribute little. If there's something you would like to know about your workshop participants, set up an intake form at registration, email them in advance, or check in with them individually in conversation or on paper when they arrive.

At the end of the workshop, you want students to feel that they have clear takeaways. Explain to them the next steps on implementing what they learned in their practice or their lives. This is where distributing a handout or pointing students toward a website is helpful. Let students know how to contact you, and follow up if appropriate with an email outlining what you covered. Know that not every studio will agree to provide email addresses to you, so you may need to get permission to ask students to sign up for a follow-up email at the end of the workshop. Have a piece of paper, tablet, or laptop ready for this.

Place Your Workshop: Inside the Studio

You might start by offering workshops at your home studio. This gives you a comfortable rookie experience: While the format may be new, the physical space and the student body will likely be familiar. In time, you might broaden your reach to offer your workshop at other studios. To do this, get a sense of the studio culture. Your masterful workshop on using props for restorative poses may not be the best fit for a hot yoga studio. And your skillful yoga for runners workshop will be preaching to the choir at a studio that already offers many weekly yoga classes geared to athletes. You want to find the sweet spot: a host studio that has a receptive student base, where your workshop will not be redundant to their current programming. If you have a friend who teaches at or studies at the location, ask them to write an email introducing you to the program director there, then follow up with a pitch.

This pitch should be a professionally written and proofread email covering:

▸ Your connection to the studio (if you had an introduction, move that liaison to BCC and thank them) or your reason for being in the area (if you have friends or family and will already be visiting, say so; this shows that you are likely not to flake out if enrollment is low)

▸ The history of the workshop's success, or your personal success as a teacher

▸ Your website address, where your reader will find a robust bio and, ideally, video clips of you teaching content similar to what you are proposing

▸ The proposed workshop title and description, and ideas about pricing

▶ A mention of your minimum, if any, and the split you would like. This could be 40:60 between teacher and venue (at major yoga centers), or 50:50 to 70:30 (elsewhere).

▶ A link to your media kit folder containing asana and headshot photos, a sample flyer, a bio, and pricing

▶ To take things to the next level, send a spreadsheet projecting how revenues will scale based on number of students. You'll need to use the formula function to do this easily—if you're not familiar, ask a friend who has facility with spreadsheets.

If you do not receive a reply, send a polite follow-up in a week.

Workshop Rates at Studios

The gold standard for experienced presenters traveling to teach workshops is 70 percent of revenue to the teacher, 30 percent to the host. This can be a percentage of gross, or of net after marketing expenses, credit card processing charges, travel fees, space rentals, and the like are subtracted out. For a newer teacher, 60:40 or 50:50 is still fair, and for teachers who travel to an established retreat center that handles most of the marketing and covers room and board, the percentage can skew even lower.

At Carolina Yoga Company, we almost exclusively offer workshops with our in-house staff. They know the studio culture and procedures well, so this is less work for us. We pay 70 percent of proceeds to the teachers when they agree to teach the workshop with no minimum number of participants. If they require a minimum, either to ensure they get a certain payment for their time (which is quite fair) or because the energetics of the workshop require a core group, we pay 50 percent to the teacher. This is because almost all of the studio's work comes in listing the workshop online and promoting it. When we need to cancel, all that work went in for no revenue.

Place Your Workshop: Outside the Studio

Some workshops naturally lend themselves to venues outside the studio setting. They could be yoga for CrossFitters held at the local CrossFit box, or yoga for knitters at the yarn shop. Or you can travel to whatever club or interest group might enjoy learning how to solve a problem or enhance their experience through yoga. You may need to handle the bulk of the contracting/terms agreement and payment processing for your host, and thus you should get a bigger split. Be sure that your insurance will extend to the venue.

Decide on When and How Long

To find the right time of year and time of day for your workshop, consider the season, any holidays, school schedules, and local events. Revisit your notes on when students encounter the problem your workshop will solve. Think about how potential students spend their weekend. If you're leading a workshop on yoga for athletic recovery, for example, it should go in the mid- to late afternoon, not on a weekend morning when people are running, riding, or playing soccer.

How long should your workshop be? It depends on the content and the students' level of experience. If students are used to sixty-minute classes, a three-hour workshop on inversions might be intimidating. Shorter would be better in this case. If you're training yoga teachers, on the other hand, a three-hour session isn't at all daunting.

Contract Your Workshop

Once you are invited to offer your workshop at the studio, you'll agree to a contract. This could be a formal document or an agreement made via email. Either way, be sure you have terms clear in writing. Your contract should outline the studio's promotion plan, your promotion plan, and how much you will be paid—including how and when. Many contracts include an agreement that some charges will come off the top before the profits are split. These can include travel, marketing fees for flyers and advertising, and credit card processing fees. Contracts should include a minimum number for enrollment, as well as a clear maximum number of enrollees or a plan for renting a larger space if needed. Outline steps for how any cancellation will be decided and announced and how and by whom refunds will be made. You can find a sample contract to copy, paste, and tweak at yogateacherhandbook.com.

At the contract stage, you'll settle on pricing for the workshop. Depending on your credentials, the topic, and the studio and local culture where you'll be teaching, this could range from $10 to $40 or more per hour of workshop time. If there is a minimum number of enrollees, implement an early-bird discount to encourage people to sign up before your do-or-die date to hit the minimum. Conversely, you can raise the price the closer you get to the workshop. However, I believe people respond well to discounts, rather than increases, which feel like late-payment penalties.

Venues may offer discounts or even full scholarship slots to their staff, space permitting. Owners generally attend free. You might want to invite a local friend to attend for free. These should be included in the contract.

Some hosts will ask you to agree to a light noncompete clause, generally by including language to the effect that you won't teach the same or a similar offering within a limited time period (like ninety days) and a limited geographical area (say, one hundred miles).

Place Your Workshop: Online

Online workshops can be hosted on your own or with a different host. If you already have a platform for online content, you could add the workshop as a stand-alone sale or part of a subscription tier. Or, your workshop may be part of a bigger event, like an online summit featuring many teachers or a platform such as Yoga International and Yoga Alliance. The split you'd receive would vary, depending on the platform.

Promote the Workshop

After working through the exercises in chapter 4, you're a whiz at promotion. Follow the steps you've learned: Generate some workshop-specific assets, plan a promotion calendar, and schedule your marketing for newsletters, social media, and, if relevant, paper.

For onetime workshops, spending a small amount on a targeted ad on Facebook or Instagram may make sense. Use the advertising tool to narrow down your audience to the exact students you've envisioned while developing the workshop, in the specific area. That will get you the most bang for your buck.

> ## Thank-You Notes
>
> It's both professional and polite to send a thank-you note after you've been a guest at another studio. This can be an email or a written note. As with any thank-you note, highlight one to three things that were especially wonderful about your experience. Then say you look forward to being back in the future.

Refine and Expand the Workshop

Just as you should do after classes, after offering a workshop, you should make notes on how it went and how you can improve in the future. It is also useful to ask students for feedback, though this may not be something you do after your regular class. Your workshop students will have a shared interest in the topic you taught on, and they may have enough experience to give you useful constructive criticism so you can improve the workshop the next time it is offered.

To gather this feedback, bring a sheet or half sheet of paper with just a few prompts on it. I favor a "keep/drop/add" trio of questions, which echoes the roses/thorns/buds model.

- ▶ Keep: What did you find most useful in this workshop?
- ▶ Drop: What was unclear or confusing?
- ▶ Add: What could be included in the future to enhance your experience?

For a onetime workshop out of your usual market, receiving anonymous feedback makes sense. If you're leading something for teachers or something that is going to have a round two in the future, you might choose to ask for student names and contact information so that you can follow up.

An alternative is to create a web form and send your students a follow-up email—maybe with an electronic version of the handout you created for the workshop—asking them to offer you feedback. Or simply ask for a reply to your email.

I favor both: a short paper evaluation at the end of the workshop, while students have the content fresh in their minds, and an electronic invitation for more feedback a few days later, when the content has been digested. This email could also invite students to offer a short testimonial for use on your website and in your workshop offerings form (see the next section).

Also ask the venue for feedback. Tell the manager or owner that you are eager to hear how you can improve, and that at any point you'd like to know the feedback that students are sharing.

Once you have this feedback, refine your offering accordingly, then work to schedule it again. You could offer it at the same venue in another season or at another venue—provided it doesn't breach your contract. As you prepare to offer the workshop again, you may need to scale it up or down. Maybe it was too long, and you want to condense. On the other hand, perhaps you can see ways to expand it, either into a weekend or into a series or a weeklong intensive or a teacher training.

Next Step: Develop a Workshop Offerings Form

As you gain experience leading workshops, and interest in booking you grows, you should develop a workshop offerings form. This document, saved as a PDF, will include many of the typical media kit assets: your headshot and other pictures, short and longer bios, a list of your social media addresses. It should also include a menu of workshops that you can offer, with descriptions that studios can imagine cutting and pasting to their website. Include a line about typical workshop length and, when relevant, ways to spin each workshop. If you are very popular, you might also include a booking rate sheet.

If your workshop offerings document is well written, studios will see the value in your offerings for their particular student base and will be able to cut and paste your description when they create the registration for the workshop. While it's good to have one generic workshop offerings form available on your website, you'll get even better traction if, after carefully researching their vibe, class and workshop offering, and student demographic, you customize the form to each studio you pitch. If you aren't physically in the area, do your research online or send a friend.

Develop a Workshop Offerings Document

Pull together a Workshop Offerings form. This document should include:

▶ A front page with a smiling picture of you, contact information, and one or two paragraphs of bio

▶ Some testimonials from well-known teachers and your students

▶ A list of workshops you can teach, each with a title, time or a time range, a robust description, props needed, and suggested pricing

▶ Your desired pay rate, including a minimum, if you have one

▶ A sample contract

Save this document in PDF format and put a copy in your media kit and on your website. You'll find my workshop offerings form at yogateacherhandbook.com.

Demand Waxes and Wanes

Even after running a studio for a decade, I still can't always put my finger on which workshops will make their minimum enrollment. Sometimes we take a chance on a workshop I think will be under-enrolled and it sells out; other times a surefire bet fizzles. Often the first iteration of an offering is huge, but a second one run a few months later won't pull the same numbers. Perhaps the first round drew all the interested students.

Know that many factors go into workshop enrollment numbers. Some of them can be quantified—the profile of the teacher, the usefulness of the content—and some are less easy to measure or to reproduce.

DEVELOPING SERIES

A *series*, as opposed to a workshop, happens more than once, generally on the same day of the week and at the same time over a series of four to twelve meetings. We've offered dozens of series at Carolina Yoga, from Yoga 101 and Flow Yoga 101 to Yoga vs. Trauma, Yoga for Athletic Recovery, and Yoga for Back Care. As the titles imply, series address a population or a special topic but go either broader or deeper than a workshop.

Series have the benefit of building progressively, so concepts or movements that are introduced in the beginning can be reinforced and revised in subsequent meetings. And series can lead to other series: Yoga 101 to Yoga 102 or Yoga 201, Basics of Acro Yoga to Intermediate Acro Yoga, etc. Once you have developed the syllabus for a series, you can repeat it year after year.

At Carolina Yoga, we offer series in both *closed* and *open* format. A closed series requires students to commit for the full run of the series, with no drop-ins allowed (they can drop out, of course). This is good for true basics, like Yoga 101, and for sensitive topics—Yoga vs. Eating Disorders, Yoga for Trauma—where the group dynamic is critical to creating a safe space for students. These workshops also require extra training on behalf of the teacher.

An open series does allow drop-ins, generally at a price that's higher than the price of a regular drop-in class. Students who drop in recognize that they are joining midstream, and that their classmates will have seen some of the concepts and movements already. But in the context of our open series, each session also works as a standalone. Think of it as an anthology series, like *Law and Order*: There is much to be gained by following the characters' arcs over a season or the run of the show, but each episode also offers a beginning, middle, and end of its own.

To accommodate the teacher's expertise and to incentivize students to commit to the full series, we pay well (70 percent of series price to the teacher if there is no minimum for the series, 50 percent if there is) and price the series appealingly. For students, committing to a four-week series can cost less than dropping in for four regular classes, but dropping in to a single session of an open series will cost more than a regular class. For example, a four-week series could be $50 or $60 ($12.50 or $15/class), but a single drop-in could be $15 or $20.

Like workshops, series can run outside the studio system. If you have a venue—a church basement or a high school gym, for example—a series is a good choice because it has clear start and end dates. Series can also run online in real time.

Envision Your Series as a Repeating Workshop

To home in on a topic, description, lesson plans, placing, and promotion strategy, follow the steps outlined in our investigation of workshops above.

One exception on how you would teach series rather than workshops: Depending on the topic and your methods, it might be useful to allow time for students to introduce themselves or to talk briefly each session about anything they've realized, noticed, or found changed since the previous week. Or create an email list, Facebook group, or group chat for your students, so they can discuss the content with each other outside class. Some online platforms will have a forum built in to course software.

TEACHING ONLINE COURSES

Removed from the constraints of time and space, your online content can take the form of single-session workshops, multi-session series, or online courses of any stripe. A course could be Yoga 101, a monthlong challenge with daily exercises, fourteen days to handstand, or continuing education for teachers—whatever best suits your interests and teaching skills. These courses may be asynchronous, or they may include a combination of students moving through lectures and practices on their own with occasional check-ins. Depending on your content and setup choices, you can release lessons to your students on a weekly basis, require they finish one (and even pass a quiz) before starting the next, or let them pick and choose how to move through the course. You may price these however you see fit. Since they take a lot of work to organize, courses are typically priced high. And since very little is required for maintenance after the initial work is done, teachers frequently offer discount codes and incentives.

Some of the platforms that you may use for your online studio are set up to handle courses—Namastream is one example—or, you can host your courses on dedicated e-learning platforms, such as Coursera, Teachable, and Udemy. A benefit is their help with promotion; a drawback is their taking a bigger cut of the revenue. Platforms like Teachable and plug-ins such as LearnDash and Sensei LMS work with a WordPress site. Visit yogateacherhandbook.com for more suggestions.

Typically, teachers progress to creating online courses after several years of experience teaching the course content in person. But in the post-COVID world, where people are more familiar with online learning, you may have success with an online course right out of the gate. If you are handy with content production and comfortable with the e-learning platform you choose, this can be a great way to earn passive income and help students you would never encounter in person. The instructions in "Content Creation" that follow will get you started.

TEACHING PRIVATE LESSONS

Some people are naturals in a private lesson: they shine in giving personalized attention to one student or a small group. Others would rather teach a full room of strangers than spend an hour one-on-one with a student. Know yourself! Teaching private lessons can be a mainstay of your yoga career if you enjoy them and you live in an area with a culture that values them, like New York City and Los Angeles. Or you may teach private lessons only rarely and at a very high price or, conversely, for free as a service to the needy or as a gift to friends and family.

Finding Private Clients

Private clients can be divided into a few groups. Knowing which of these you want to teach will help you market to them. One is the student who wants to confirm they are flexible enough to make it through your regular class without feeling embarrassed. These may be onetime gigs, but they convert to regular students in your group class. You may draw these clients from your class or through word of mouth.

Another kind of client is the student who's attended a few classes and wants individual attention for a specific goal like "I want to workshop my downward-facing dog" or "I want to make it into handstand eventually and need to learn the progressive steps to get there." In this case, instead of offering one-offs, tell potential clients what they can gain by committing to a series of five, ten, or twenty private sessions. It's a chance to customize a practice and see really targeted, tangible progress. To gain these clients, with your studio's permission, you can mention in class that you are available for private lessons to workshop particular roadblocks or build to goals.

Some private clients are well-off and because of their work schedule—or, in some cases, their fame—can't make it in to the studio. For these clients, a private lesson can look a whole lot like a very small group class, though naturally with specialized and individual attention. Word of mouth is a usual way to gain these clients. Again, you can mention in class that you do such work, and you may reach these clients through their networks. Or partner with a personal trainer or boutique gym: Approach them to say that you're available for private lessons. Offer the trainer or gym a onetime free lesson so they can see what happens in a private session with you, then ask them to talk it up to their clients.

Some bookings will be for a special occasion, like a family reunion, a bridal shower, or a bachelorette party. These can be a blast. Fill your lesson plan with safe but showy Instagrammable partner yoga, theme it around love, create a playlist of the bride's favorite songs, and follow the service industry's conventional wisdom: The price of anything labeled *wedding* automatically doubles. Partner with wedding planners, reception halls, and bridal shops to get out the word that you are available. Having a pretty flyer or a mention on a wedding industry website can bring these clients to you.

Pricing and Policies

People value what they pay for. If a private lesson with you costs more than a class or a private lesson with your colleagues, students will take it more seriously, turn up more reliably, and do any homework you assign more diligently. This increases the value of yoga—you already value it, obviously, and pricing it accordingly encourages your students to value it. When you charge a fair but high fee for private lessons, you will have more resources to *give* lessons away to those who would really benefit from it but can't afford it. As much as we value yoga, it is a luxury. We can't argue that it's a necessity like food or shelter; you aren't engaging in price gouging by setting a high rate. You're contributing to the economic wellness of the profession. Pricing yourself too low, on the other hand, both devalues yoga and undercuts your colleagues who also offer private lessons.

We tell our teacher trainees that $75 for an hour-long private lesson should be their minimum fresh out of training. This is about in line with massage rates; if it seems low or high to you, research massage rates in your area and align with them. Be sure also to look at your colleagues' rates, or ask them about their rates. Any professional would be willing to tell you. Say, "I'm starting to offer private lessons, and I want to make sure I'm not underselling yoga or myself. Since you have a few more years' experience than I do, I'd like to make sure I'm pricing correctly relative to you. What do you charge?"

For every year of experience, try scaling up by $5 to $10 on your base rate, so that by your fifth year you are at $100, $125, or more per hour. It is better to be too expensive than too cheap. You can always lower your rate or offer discounts, calling them "sliding scale" or "scholarships." If you mention your $75 rate to a client who then says, "That's it? I thought it would be more," you can't splutter, "I mean, $150 an hour!" And you can't raise your rates that often. Once a year or every other year is reasonable, unless you are extremely busy, or you want to cull your client list.

Decide whether you will charge a flat rate or scale your rates, so that a lesson for one to three people is, for example, $75, and every person over three is $15 more per hour. Work to find a sweet spot where the group pays only slightly more per session than they would if they came to a drop-in class.

Make your pricing obvious on your website, unless you're intentionally if-you-have-to-ask-you-can't-afford-it expensive. (You certainly shouldn't be that expensive right out of teacher training!) Have a clearly labeled page on your website describing what you offer in a private lesson and how to book. When you get a query, be sure to point your potential client to that page even if you think they've already seen it. This begins to establish student expectations about what does and doesn't happen in a private lesson. And it's a way of discussing the money without having to say it out loud, which is often difficult for yoga teachers. Either way, make sure your pricing is clear to your student.

When you are very busy or if you can't remember the last time you adjusted your rates, it's time to raise them. Decide when to implement the change: The first of the year or the first of a month are both good times. You might choose to announce your raise a month or a few weeks in advance, to encourage existing clients to buy a package at the current rates. Make the statement clearly and without apology, either in person, in writing in a frame at your checkout area (if you teach from home, this might be by the chairs where clients put on their shoes), or online. Say something like, "As of January 1, new rates for private lessons will be as follows: $100 per hour, $450 for a five-session package; $800 for a ten-session package. It's an honor to work with you to include yoga as part of your self-care plan!"

Students who can't afford the new pricing will let you know. At that point, you can choose to grandfather them in at the old rate or refer them to a colleague who charges less.

If you are affiliated with a studio, your studio might handle booking private lessons for you, and would then take a cut. This could be up to 50 percent of the cost of the lesson. Such studios would not want you soliciting their students for private lessons offsite, so be very clear on what the studio policy is.

Determine the best way to book lessons—phone calls, emails, or scheduling software, which can be as simple as using a Google calendar and its invitations feature. At your first contact with the student, explain your cancellation policy. I suggest announcing that you charge for cancellations within 24 hours, except in the case of true emergency or sudden illness. If you confirm appointments either manually or automatically, using a scheduled email or scheduling software, you'll likely never have to implement your charge-for-cancellation policy.

Use an intake form that starts with a waiver and continues to a questionnaire about what your student would like to learn, as well as their goals. If their goals aren't clear, use a series of poses to observe their strengths and imbalances, then strategize about how you can address these imbalances. Take baseline measurements: how long your student can hold tree, where they are in downward dog, or where their hands wind up in cow-face arms. You'll then be able to track progress as you work together. Take some before pictures, or record a short video.

You'll need a method to take payment—if you are running a credit card, be prepared with an app like Square or Stripe open, logged in, and ready to go. You might like to take payment at the start of the lesson, which gets what might feel like an uncomfortable transaction out of the way. Or take it at the end, which is also a good time to schedule the next lesson. If you offer multi-lesson packages, develop a way to keep track of how many sessions your clients have left. A notes file or your calendar app can help.

Add Value

Private lessons can very specifically target the challenges and needs of the student where a regular class cannot. Add value on top of this by continuing the personalization in ways that would be tough to do for a whole class. Start with a follow-up email or handout with notes about what you worked on and any takeaways. You might assign homework, or record a sequence for your student to follow along with in the days between lessons.

If you are confident with physical assists and have your student's express permission, you will have a lot more time to offer them in a private lesson. Be careful not to give so many assists that you either make the client too reliant on your touch or leave them feeling scrutinized.

Another way to add value to lessons with your longtime clients is to slowly amass a prop closet for them. If you travel to your client, you could bring a few different mats for a "test drive," then give them (or sell them) a mat in their favorite material and thickness. Pick up a pair of blocks or straps, make them a feature in your next few lessons, and leave them at the client's house as part of their yoga props cabinet. You could even mark anniversaries with such a gift, or throw in a mat or some props when clients buy a long-term class package: Buy twenty lessons, get a bolster.

Where to Meet

The studio is usually the best place to meet in person. It has the benefit of all the props, and it's neutral ground. If—and only if—you are confident in your safety, you can travel to a client's home for a lesson. Since this adds convenience for your client, consider adding a travel fee to your rates. This could be $10 to cover your gas or the cost of public transportation, or it could be half the hourly rate for the lesson itself to cover travel time. You get to decide! If you are in a student's home, seek to reduce distractions: Ask them to turn off their ringer, put the dog outside, or send the kids out of the house, when feasible. Wear a watch so you can keep track of the time.

If you are very confident in your own safety, you can have clients visit you for a private lesson. In this case, you'll have your props handy and be able to control the environment for sound, lighting, temperature, and so on. Be sure to issue clear parking instructions to your client and to have a clean, well-stocked bathroom available, as well as a clear view of a clock or your watch while you teach.

If you are giving private lessons online, see what platform your student prefers; this reduces technical problems and makes the experience easiest for your student. Face-Time, Skype, and Google Hangouts all work fine. Be clear whether they should call you or you should call them at the appointed time. Do your intake form and waiver ahead of time via email. Since you will not be on-hand with props, ask what equipment is available to your student, or plan a prop-free lesson. Ask for payment before the session begins, unless you know the student quite well. One benefit of virtual private lessons is that they can be recorded, if you and your student both agree. In that case, aim to use a platform that allows for easy recording, like Skype. FaceTime calls can be recorded using Quick-Time, but it's not as easy. Having a recording adds good value to the lesson!

Scouting Visit

Before your first session, whether for a studio class, workshop, private lesson, or one-off promotional or volunteer event, try to pay a scouting visit whenever possible. As you do, take stock of all the variables we explored in chapter 7. What's the temperature, and can you change it? What's the sound like? Will you use music, and if so, how will you work it? Will you use a microphone, and if so, how will you work it? What's the lighting situation, and how can you adjust it? Where will you set up? What props will students have handy? If you'll be holding class outside, do this visit at the same time of day you'll be teaching during the event, because different lighting can really affect students' experience. For outdoor venues, consider what you will do in case of rain: move indoors or online, postpone, or cancel. In the latter cases, how will you announce this decision, and how will you issue refunds? Thinking through all of these contingencies before the actual session will ease your mind and free your energy to teach your students to the best of your ability. If you can't show up on a separate scouting visit, arrive super early so you can make smart choices to offer students the best possible experience.

TEACHING CORPORATE CLASSES

A variation on the private lesson is a standing corporate class, where you travel to an office, a hotel, or an apartment building—or to a virtual platform—to offer a weekly or monthly session to employees, clients, or residents. You'll plan this like a class or, if it happens less frequently or students have no experience, a workshop.

Your studio may connect you with corporate clients. In this case, they may take a onetime finder's fee or a regular cut of the class, especially if they process payment. If you would like to solicit such classes for yourself, construct an email following the advice above for pitching a workshop. Send it to wellness managers and property managers with an explanation of how yoga will enhance employees' well-being or productivity, or how having yoga as an amenity will make a hotel or apartment building more attractive to guests or renters.

To price these classes, figure out who is paying. Is it the business whose location you're visiting? You might price it at your private-lesson rate, perhaps with some travel time added. Is it the students themselves, either completely or as a supplement to a base rate from the company? If so, set your prices so that you will get the equivalent of your private-lesson rate or higher.

It's smart to set a range of dates to see if this is a good fit for the business, the students, and you. A month of trial classes should be enough to test the waters. Then you can extend the contract, renegotiate it, or let it go.

Be sure that you have a trusted substitute teacher on deck to cover these classes if you have an emergency. Have them totally up to speed on the class: where it's held and when, as well as how to get there, where to park, and whether and how to take payment. Bringing your sub along when you teach to see everything firsthand and meet the students is a smart move. Also ensure that you have a clear way to announce any class cancellations on account of illness or weather, or weeks off for holidays or travel.

FREE CLASSES AT STORES

You may have noticed that retail stores selling yoga clothing often host weekly classes. These attract practitioners, who spend an hour or more in the company of the clothes, with the idea that they are more likely to buy. In my experience—and I would be happy to be wrong here!—in-store classes do not convert to paying students at the studio. Who comes to free classes at the mall? People who know they can get free yoga there every week!

You might have your own reasons for saying yes to an invitation to lead a free in-store class. Maybe you're offered an outfit in exchange for your time—this could be a good deal, coming to the equivalent of $200 for an hour of your time. Or maybe you want to gain experience as a new teacher, or even apply for a job in the store. Be clear about your reasons. Just don't expect the students, who may be very nice, to follow you to the studio or a private lesson. That doesn't mean you can't try!

If you are teaching a free class, plan to attend the class sometime in the weeks before it's your turn to teach it. Look at the students, gauge their experience level and needs, and figure out how you can best use the space and your time. Decide how you can offer students something of value, both in your lesson plan and in exchange for signing up for your newsletter. Confirm with the venue that you can collect email addresses, then at the end of your class, invite students to sign up to receive a video, or a coupon for a discounted class with you elsewhere, whatever you think will make the best incentive.

FUNDRAISER CLASSES AND DONATIONS

One way to use your teaching skill for good is to offer a fundraiser or donation class for a charitable cause. This could be something you do annually, like a class for the food bank offered every Thanksgiving. Or it could be a response to a natural disaster, like a hurricane.

For such a class, you could either suggest a donation or sell "tickets," proceeds from which are donated. The latter may be easier if you can run it through a studio or a service like Eventbrite. Check with the studio owner and your accountant about how to log these. If you are asking students for a donation at the class, set out a box for cash or check donations, which you'll then pass directly along to the charity. Or set up a tablet or laptop with the charity's site open so people can make credit card donations. If you're raising money for a local charity, ask if they could send a staff member to come say a few words at the start of class. This direct appeal will personalize the ask and is likely to generate more donations.

You might also offer a private lesson or a series of three or five classes as an incentive at a silent auction for a cause you believe in. Often, bidders at these auctions intend to take the class or lesson but never actually follow through. If people do follow through, they are likely to already be existing customers of your business. Either way, the charity will have benefited, and you'll have put your name in front of people who have the means and the heart to attend charity events. Ask your accountant how to factor this donation in to your tax records.

Beyond your offerings at your home studio and in your local area, you might connect far outside the studio setting. This could be at a retreat, at yoga festivals, or through the content you generate.

RETREATS

A yoga retreat is a bucket-list item for many practitioners, combining their love of yoga with a fun weekend or week of travel. If you're interested in leading retreats, give your interest some serious thought. What is your ideal retreat experience, both for yourself and for your students? How you prepare for these depends on your vision: Are you taking existing students on a fun vacation with some yoga thrown in? Are you partnering with an established retreat center to offer advanced trainings for serious students, or continuing education to yoga teachers? Are students going to leave feeling like they had a fun break, or like they've undergone deep personal transformation?

If you are leading a retreat on your own, you'll have all the contingencies of setting up your own workshop—booking the space, supplying the props, marketing the event, processing payments, establishing a clear refund policy—in addition to playing cruise director for your students. This can quickly become overwhelming. To maximize the experience for both you and your students, it can be wise to partner with one or more teachers or event coordinators so that you focus only on what you're good at. That also takes some of the work off you so that you can enjoy the trip yourself. Bringing a social director, a logistics coordinator, even a chef, will reduce your personal obligation while adding value for your students.

If you are in charge of the retreat, whether you're bringing your own staff or using one on location, take plenty of time to strategize how you will control the smooth movement of your group from start to finish. Will you cover airport transfers to your destination? How will students move around once they're at the destination? If you are hiring a driver, how will you confirm they are licensed and insured? How and when will students eat? What activities will you offer in addition to yoga? It's good to present a range of choices, but be sure also to build in downtime and flex time.

There are many international retreat centers that cover much of the logistics, freeing you up to teach yoga. A quick internet search will turn these up. Ask lots of questions, and be sure to ask for references from former teachers and their students. What looks incredible online might not be so wonderful in person—and vice versa. Any reputable center will be happy to give you references, and some of them will invite you for a brief stay so that you can assess whether it's a good fit for you and your student base. As you gain a profile as a teacher, you'll find retreat centers reaching out to sell themselves to you. Keep your eyes on the prize: What is *your* vision for your retreat? Just because a particular center wants you doesn't mean it's the ideal fit.

Beyond vacation-style retreats are programs you might offer at established yoga retreat centers, like Kripalu, the Omega Institute, 1440 Multiversity, the Mount Madonna Center, and Esalen. When you teach at such a center, you'll be responsible only for your teaching hours and off the clock the rest of the time. You might choose to engage with your students at meals, or in study sessions, or not. If you are an introvert or a business owner with other work to attend to each day, the ample downtime you'll be able to carve out at an established center is priceless. Retreat centers generally do good promotion, as well, helping you reach students who wouldn't find you otherwise, and whom you can then funnel into your other offerings. (Each year, I draw one or two students from Kripalu to North Carolina to take our teacher trainings.) In exchange, of course, you'll be getting paid a smaller cut of the proceeds from your program.

If you're interested in teaching at such places, dig in on their websites. Each should outline how to "pitch" a program. Ask your yoga mentors if they have any connections that might pull you to the top of the application pile—as with many things, who you know is as important as what you know, and one well-placed recommendation can open doors for you. Once you are a regular presence at one center, programmers at other centers are more likely to recognize your name and to consider you for their locations.

FESTIVALS

Eventually, you may be invited to teach (or apply to teach) at a yoga festival. These can be big corporate events like Wanderlust, or more homegrown (Asheville Yoga Festival, Floyd Yoga Jam). This can be a fun weekend and a chance to meet new students and colleagues. Don't expect to be paid a ton—but do expect to have fun!

Like many things in the professional world, these festivals rely on networks and word of mouth to make their hiring decisions. Cold calls can work, for sure, but your best way in will be focusing on being a demonstrably good teacher with a visible presence online, both with content to share—videos, articles, social media posts—and a quantifiable following. Let your mentors know you're looking to teach at festivals; they may be able to make some introductions for you.

When you are invited to a festival, you'll be asked to submit descriptions of your workshops. Start with the workshops you've been teaching, and consider the needs of the festival participants. Are they looking for challenge? Are the majority of offerings already challenging, in which case you can offer a mellow or restorative class? Festivals are a chance to explore special topics, like yoga hybrids, partner yoga, yoga with live music, chakra balancing, and so on.

Make it clear in your contract whether the festival is paying for your travel, whether you receive a per diem to cover food, and what your accommodations will be. When you are a newer teacher, your contract will have fewer perks. When you're so busy that you need to turn down some invitations, you should begin to ask for more accommodations in the form of single rooms, airport transfers, on-site transportation, and so on.

Be sure that you have a capture device to help students connect with you and continue the relationship beyond the festival itself, just as you have developed for off-site classes and workshops. This could be offering a copy of your playlist to students who sign up for your newsletter, encouraging people to follow you on Instagram to see a video of the peak sequence you taught, or pointing people to online video classes with you. It's usually easiest to offer a piece of free content in exchange for an email address.

As you would after a workshop, write a thank-you message to the festival organizers. Ask for their feedback about your offerings, and let them know that you are eager to be invited back. You can say something like, "Thank you for having me, I had a great time! X, Y, and Z were especially well done. If I were lucky enough to be invited back in the future, what would you like me to change?"

Yoga Agents

There are a few outfits that might like to represent you, for a fee. These could be yoga talent agencies or broader talent agencies like Creative Artists Agency (CAA). If you feel like you're busy enough to need an agent to help you find the best outlets for your teaching, ask your yoga mentors for recommendations. Good agents are worth their weight in gold. They create opportunities for you and ensure that your contracts are skewed in your favor. Good agents will easily pay for themselves. A bad agent will promise you the moon and never deliver. If someone approaches you offering representation, do your due diligence. Ask for references and follow up with them. Before you sign a contract, review it carefully and be clear on your options for severing ties. Generally, an agent who brokers a client connection for you will be entitled to a cut—often 15 percent—of all work you do with that client in perpetuity.

CONTENT CREATION

What is this "content" that will help students connect with you? It's something of value that will help students feel better through yoga. It could be as simple as an inspiring quote, or a brief description of a pose or an exercise or as complex as a video series, online class library, or an ebook. There are only so many hours in a day you can interact with students in person, and those hours are tied to one physical location. Creating and sharing content will help your students find connection when you aren't physically present.

Early in my career, I used my experience with writing to offer a pose-of-the-month column in my statewide endurance sports magazine. The audience was clear: runners, cyclists, and triathletes. The problem they had was also clear: sport-specific tightness that might lead to imbalances, coupled with a general inability to relax. Each month, I outlined the what, when, why, and how of a particular pose or breath exercise to solve these problems. Then I collected some of the pose images into a slideshow, recorded a voice track describing how to do them, and posted these recordings as a podcast, Sage Yoga Training. Eventually I had a catalog of a dozen or so of these, which I was able to reference when I pitched the book that became *The Athlete's Guide to Yoga*. On the strength of the book, I was hired to write articles and blog posts for *Runner's World* and *Yoga Journal*. Later still I partnered with Yoga Vibes to record my classes for athletes and post them online, so that people could follow along with a video class to help them balance themselves with yoga.

All of this is content—articles, podcasts, books, and videos. My content generation started with my genuine interest in yoga for endurance athletes, capitalized on my studies in writing and my experience in radio production, took advantage of my husband's ability with a digital camera, and grew from short snippets into content across a number of media: written, audio, and video.

What Do You Have to Say?

Creating content follows many of the steps you learned for planning a workshop. You need to figure out a way to help people through yoga. This could be by thinking of specialized activities or occupations, then thinking of a problem or a goal they have and how yoga can solve it or help them reach it. You can then start to think about where and how you might share this content. Here are a pair of exercises to get you thinking.

Find Your Message and Your Platform

Respond to these prompts.

- ▶ When do you feel most helpful as a teacher? Why? Where does this happen?
- ▶ What's your favorite group to lead in a yoga practice? Why? What do these people all have in common? That is, who are your students?
- ▶ What is a problem they have?
- ▶ Where does that problem arise?

▶ When does that problem emerge?

▶ Why does that problem happen?

▶ How can they deploy your solution? What are the steps? Lay them out in detail.

▶ What will they wind up with when the problem is solved?

▶ Who is your message for? Who is it *not* for? How can those it is not for adapt it, or find a solution to their unique problems?

Next, ask yourself these questions and note your answers.

▶ Who/what are the thought leaders in your niche? How do they communicate?

▶ Where does your audience meet: online? in person?

▶ What are your strengths and production talents/resources as a writer/artist/teacher?

▶ What tools do you already have to get started?

Your response is now the basis for an article or a blog post, or for a short video. If it isn't short, you can make it into a series.

Content Helps Everyone

Your content doesn't just help your students, although that is the number one reason to create and share it. It will also get you attention and open doors for you. Many of my most rewarding career connections, from my years of sponsorship by prAna to teaching on the Wanderlust circuit, came because I had a body of work that people found useful.

Plan Your Content

To home in further on your message, clearly define the problem and the steps to solving it with yoga. What will your readers or viewers wind up with when the problem is solved: more comfortable hamstrings, better ability to meditate, or a good night's sleep? Who is your message for, and who is it *not* for?

Once you're clear on these answers, you can outline your content. Start with an introduction that is as explicit as you can be to define the problem. Then list your solution step by step, point by point. As you go, start to list what photos, videos, or other illustrations might help. This will become your asset list.

Now set yourself a timeline. You'll need to work in three categories: planning your content, which you've already begun; producing it; and promoting it. For each of these, write out each next step to take. Set concrete dates by which you will take these steps, and find a way to build in some accountability: Work with a friend and promise to review each other's material at a scheduled meeting, for example.

Make an Outline and Timeline

Start an outline of your content by responding to these prompts.

▸ Write an introduction defining the problem and pointing to the solution. Be as explicit as you can.

▸ List the steps of the solution point by point.

▸ Begin to note what photos/video might help.

Draft a timeline:

Planning
1. List the first step (e.g., type out an outline and shot list)
2. And the next one after that
3. Etc.

Production
1. List the first step (e.g., line up a photographer)
2. And the next one after that
3. Etc.

Promotion
1. List the first step (e.g., add a blog to your website)
2. And the next one after that
3. Etc.

Produce and Place Your Content

Now it's time to put your plan into action. Whether you are working alone or with a photographer or videographer, schedule your writing or shooting time as an appointment. Accept some discomfort and procrastination as part of the writing process—and just get started. As you do, capture everything that comes to mind on your topic; you can edit it later.

There's nothing new under the sun. Much of what you have to say has already been said by others before you. There are only so many ways to move a body, so many uses for props, so many ways to explain the chakras. Recognize, though, that no one has done it exactly the way you have. Focus on what makes you unique, with special attention to the audience you're writing for. The clearer you can keep your vision of who you're talking to, the easier it will be to create fresh and useful content, even if you're covering something seemingly "basic," like how to do mountain pose.

Both for writing and for imagery, you'll need to find the right tone and look. Looking at role models can be helpful here. Once you've decided on a filter, a writing style, or a standard introduction and closing to your videos, make notes about it so you can deploy it in future episodes of the series.

Where you place your content is up to you. Some or all of these platforms may be especially exciting to you—choose the ones that excite you, instead of forcing yourself to work in a medium that you find difficult.

Social media. Social media is a friendly starting point for many, as you may already be offering pose tutorials or inspirational quotes there. Social media captions now count as writing—you can share something extremely useful in even a few sentences, especially when it's accompanied by a photo or video. Including such captions also makes your content more accessible to the visually impaired.

Use a common set of hashtags every time you post. One or two of these hashtags should be very specific to your unique content, and the rest can be slightly broader, so you can expand your reach to people who are searching by tag.

DIY writing online. If you enjoy writing, you can post your content to a blog hosted on your own site. Promote it with social media posts that pull a short tidbit out of your longer writing. Each blog post can be one to five paragraphs long. If you're writing more than that, divvy it up into a series of posts, published a week apart.

Down the road, you can collect your blog posts into an ebook (you can do this on your own using various online outfits, including Amazon Kindle Direct Publishing), or eventually into a print book. Either would provide a passive income stream.

Other sites online. You can pitch your article to an online site that specializes in yoga or movement topics. With many magazines closing or moving away from print and into online spaces, there's usually not much money to be earned by placing an article. Instead, use the opportunity to expand your profile. Be sure your article contains a rich biography with links for readers to follow you online, and an incentive to visit your site and learn more—possibly in a paid video series.

Free video online. It's easy to share content on social media—just go live and talk about how to solve a problem with yoga! You can also record and edit videos for YouTube or other online sites where viewers can access them for free. Follow the video advice you'll find in chapter 7.

DIY premium video online. As we saw at the beginning of this chapter, you can create your own virtual yoga studio housing a library of tutorials and classes. If you are catching seasonal visitors, this is another way to connect with your students once they leave town. You might eventually do some or all of your teaching online, which has the added benefit of being asynchronous: You do not have to appear in person at a set time, and the number of hours you could be teaching per week scales from five to twenty or so, to become infinite.

Established yoga streaming sites. In time, you might contribute classes to a high-profile site that will film them, sell them, and pass you a cut of the proceeds. The field of such sites is constantly changing, but you might look at Yoga Vibes, Alo, Glo, or OmStars. Just as in booking studio classes, there's a chicken-and-egg conundrum here. It can be tough to develop the follower base to bring you to the notice of the big platforms, which might not want to take a chance on you without a proven track record.

To get out of this vicious cycle, share snippets of your content widely and freely. This doesn't mean it all needs to be free, but you could cut a one- to three-minute video out of a longer one and offer the short one free. Be sure it contains a useful lesson and leaves viewers wanting to upgrade to the full-length video. The more you focus on genuinely helping people with your content, the more opportunities you'll have to share it with a wider audience.

Videoconferencing live classes. During the COVID-19 pandemic, many studios encouraged their teachers to lead live classes over videoconferencing software. Teachers were paid either by the studio or directly by students. This served as a bridge to keep students connected with their favorite local teachers and, for the studios, to provide value for those paying for the recurring memberships that sustain them. Now that students are familiar with such platforms as a viable way to do yoga, they are an option when teacher and students can't be together in the same room at the same time. Since teaching live-stream classes requires much more demonstration on the part of the teacher, online instruction is no more (and possibly far less) sustainable than teaching the same schedule in person. Compound these demands with the number of technical issues that could occur—from Internet slowness to security violations—and multiply it by the sheer volume of other people offering the same thing, and you'll find it's not an appealing long-term solution. I suggest you prioritize creating *asynchronous* content like a library of online classes available by rental fee or subscription. This maximizes the potential amount you can earn without putting demands on you to be in a particular place at a particular time with a particular set of tech specs. That way, you can earn money without needing to commit yourself to a schedule.

Strategize Your Content

Since you can branch in so many different directions as you produce useful content, the direction you choose to go will dictate your next steps. If you are excited about one or more ideas, take a moment to jot down what they are, where you'll place them, who might be able to help you, and what your first next steps are toward fulfilling your vision.

The Funnel

When you share content in any medium, include a robust bio that serves as a funnel to keep your audience connected to you. Issue a call to action, such as, "Come to my site at sagerountree.com to find videos and books about how to find better balance with yoga." As readers browse your site, they should be invited to sign up for your newsletter with another call to action: "Sign up for the newsletter and you'll get a code to watch a premium video for free." Every interaction has rewarding information *and* a way to stay connected and learn more.

Promote Your Content

Promotion of your content works much like promoting a workshop or any other offering: You'll schedule a promotion calendar and, when possible, automate it. Naturally, the content you make will go into your newsletter! Here's some specialized advice about content promotion.

Tease your content. Outline the problem that you've identified and tease that you have the solution—and it will be available when readers click here, or viewers press play, or folks order your book. Get your audience excited to learn from you the solution to the problem.

Share and repurpose your content. Most content is evergreen, meaning it is relevant anytime. You can usually take a point or two out of your writing—maybe your first or second paragraph—and use them to promote the bigger piece of writing. Or grab thirty seconds to a minute from a shorter video so viewers have a sense of what they're committing to if they watch the whole thing.

Sometimes you can take an image or a video you've used to make one point and repurpose it to make a new point. Be on the lookout for ways to spin your old content in fresh ways.

Journalists and Publicity

As you develop a niche and a platform, you might have journalists reach out to you as an expert. Usually they'll send you an email or a direct message (which you can then move to email) with their article topic and a few prompts for quotes. You can then respond in writing or with a phone call. Just as you would in class, you'll find yourself saying the same thing over and over—and that's not only OK, it's good. Each press contact is a chance to reach a broader base of students who likely haven't heard your message yet. When you give an interview, add a link to your file on publicity you've had, and share the finished product on your social media and in your newsletter.

Evaluation and Replication

As with your weekly classes and any workshop you teach, you should regularly assess your content to see how it landed with your audience. If you've published online, you should have access to statistics in the form of page views or link clicks (you can get these from Google Analytics or other stat-counting programs) or likes and saves and comments on social media.

Assess what your audience found useful and what they found confusing. Then plan more content based on what your audience is telling you they need.

As you gain a platform and own a niche, look for ways to collaborate with others with similar or complementary skills. You might partner with one or more colleagues to run an Instagram challenge, or coauthor some writing—or devise an in-person workshop that plays to your combined strengths. Having the right partner can excite you about your content all over again. When you have the right collaborator, it feels like you do less than half the work for more than twice the fun.

As you continue to create content through the years, be sure to catalog it so your students can connect with your work, both recent and older. This could mean updating your website regularly to keep links fresh or restructuring it so students can find what they are looking for.

For more on creating content and detailed instructions on how to plan, place, and promote your content, please take the Content Workshop at sageyogateachertraining.com.

SPONSORSHIPS

Once you are generating quality content—even just well-done social media posts— brands may seek you out to offer partnerships and sponsorships. This could be as small as free product in the hopes that you'll mention it or give a review, or as big as being paid for a post or salaried as a brand ambassador. You will also be offered advice on promoting your social media or guest blog posts. You might find yourself inundated with these; it's OK to ignore them if they don't align with your vision for your career.

If you are paid to promote a product on social media—even if the payment is receiving the product itself—you should make that clear in your post with a hashtag like #ad, or #sponsoredpost, whatever the platform requires. But you don't want to stretch your students' goodwill thin by constantly shilling to them. When you're recommending a product simply because you love it, make that clear, too! Both your students and that brand (tag them!) will appreciate your genuine praise.

If a brand invites you to be an ambassador, be clear on what that means. In general, they will expect a certain number of in-store appearances or social media posts each month. While it's exciting to feel wanted, be sure you believe in the brand and think carefully about whether they are offering you enough to use their product to the exclusion of other comparable products you own. For example, if a clothing company wants you to wear their clothes exclusively, you need to receive enough of the clothes that it won't be a difficult thing to do.

DISCOUNTS

Once you are a Yoga Alliance–registered teacher or have a regular class, or both, you might be eligible for discounts at clothing stores like lululemon athletica and Athleta. Ask at the counter, and be prepared to show a business card, give your Yoga Alliance registry number, or demonstrate that you are a regular teacher at a local studio. These discounts are generally meant for you and you alone. The idea is that you will wear the discounted items you buy when you teach. Discounts are not to be used to buy gifts for friends, unless permission is expressly granted. Some companies let affiliates buy gifts before the holidays. Be sure to ask instead of violating the terms of the discount.

You can create your own opportunities as well. If there's a brand you'd like to have a discount on, it doesn't hurt to ask! Reach out with enthusiastic praise and see if they have a pro discount or might create one for you. Having statistics about your follower base, like its size or your email newsletter list, your follower count, and so on, will help make your case.

This is exactly the kind of hustle you'll need to demonstrate if you want to make yoga a full-time job.

11

Making Yoga Your Full-Time Job

· ·

A LUCKY FEW PEOPLE make yoga a full-time job. I wouldn't even strictly count myself among them, as some of my income is from my ownership of other businesses, and I count on my husband's benefits for my health insurance.

How will you know when you're ready to make the move to being a full-time or almost full-time yoga teacher? You won't. If you waited until you were completely ready, you'd never start! But you'll feel more excited about the possibilities than scared about what might not work out.

Since you won't be literally teaching yoga forty hours a week, making it a full-time job means you need *several* revenue streams. This is not just classes, not just private lessons—and not just things you do in person. This is why monetized asynchronous online content matters. Even if you were earning a good living traveling the world, teaching workshops a dozen weekends of the year, you'd want a diverse set of income streams, since one deep vein thrombosis or bad inner-ear infection preventing you from air travel could wipe out your annual pay.

Even if teaching full-time isn't your goal, it's smart to find ways to diversify your offerings. Don't put all your eggs in one basket that depends upon your body holding up, especially if you teach a very physically demanding form of yoga or movement. Move some of your eggs into other baskets, like teaching meditation, training teachers, and other, less physical pursuits.

Set Your Vision

If you think you'd one day like to go all in on yoga as your primary source of income, whether you're still looking at teacher trainings or feeling fed up with your day job, take some time first to dream and then to have a clear-eyed look at whether your dreams will stand up to reality. These prompts will help; write a little in response to each. Then talk about what you wrote with your partner, a parent, an adult child, a good friend, your mentor, your therapist, your life coach, or any trusted counselor. Don't forget to include an accountant on this list!

▶ If you didn't need the money, how would you spend your days?

▶ If you knew you would get a *yes*, what would you ask for in your current yoga-related work? What about other local opportunities? National and international opportunities? If you were sure to succeed, what would you reach for?

▶ When in your yoga workday are you happiest? What pays your soul the biggest dividends?

▶ What part of your yoga workweek pays you the most money per hour?

▶ Is there dissonance or harmony between your answers to the two previous questions? If the former, what could you change?

▶ How much do you need to earn to cover your expenses? How much do you need to earn to cover your expenses and contribute to short-term emergency-fund savings and long-term retirement savings?

▶ What is the difference between where you are and where you need to be?

▶ What real-world opportunities can you seize or create to bridge that gap?

How I Left My Day Job

In the later years of my PhD studies, I did some freelance proofreading and copyediting for Duke University Press. As I was graduating, my wonderful supervisor there—one of the champions of my career, because his belief in me, which he expressed freely, gave me critical self-confidence—offered me a part-time job in-house, overseeing others doing the freelance work I'd been doing. After seven years of graduate school, with no appealing academic jobs to be found, I was happy to take the work, since it especially suited me as a new mother. I spent eighteen happy months working twenty—then eventually thirty—hours a week in a chic office in a renovated tobacco warehouse in downtown Durham.

What changed and led me back out of the office job? I did the math, at my husband's behest. As a part-timer, I wasn't receiving benefits—and happily, I didn't need them. And once I factored in the childcare, the gasoline and car expenses to commute, one or two lunches out, a new skirt and a new lipstick every month, my paycheck was gone. What I realized when I saw it on paper was that I was working just to fund the lifestyle of working. This suited my ego: It was a very good job in a field related to my degree, and going from graduate school to not working would have been crushing. But once I realized I could revert to freelancing and make more money, the choice was clear, if not easy. (It's so hard to quit when you have a great boss!) Once I was freelancing, it was easy to make month-by-month adjustments: I'd take more or fewer projects depending on what else was going on. Quickly, it was a second pregnancy and parenting two young daughters, then taking yoga teacher training, then transitioning to a yoga career. I recognize the immense privilege I have. And I bow to the math. The figures didn't lie: Staying in that office job wasn't smart. I hope when you look at the math, it guides you to a wise choice.

STRIKING A SMART BALANCE LOCALLY

Balance is the key across all levels. If you're going to be a full-time teacher in your local market, consider whether it is wisest to go all in at one studio, perhaps as their lead teacher, manager, or teacher trainer, or if it would be smart to have a combination of clients across a schedule that includes many studios, gyms, and private lessons. Going all in at one place, especially if it's a bigger business or a regional or national chain, may mean you get health insurance, vacation time, and other benefits of being a full-time employee.

It also means that your work is dependent on the health of that business, so consider its longevity and financial stability as you weigh any full-time job offer.

As you envisioned your ideal schedule in chapter 6, here you'll want to carefully weigh the pros and cons as you consider your practical schedule. Write out what you earn at each venue, along with hourly payments and the amount of time spent traveling.

Think about your brand and your audience. Where are your students? Are they at senior living facilities, in which case you should travel to them? Are they private clients who value yoga in their homes and pay accordingly? Or do your students travel to you? Do you have a sizable online following, or would you like to build one?

BEING A TRAVELING TEACHER

Traveling to lead workshops and to teach at festivals seems pretty glamorous from the outside. But in reality, it's a lot like being a rock star: You spend a lot of your time tied up in the logistics of getting from point A to point B (and trying to find a salad there!), where you'll deliver the same playlist to a different crowd day in and day out. This can drive you to staleness, and as a response you may wind up trying to build on what you said the previous weekend in an attempt to keep yourself intellectually stimulated. But the students in the new town need to hear the basics again. Remember: You're the only one who's ever heard every word you say.

When you travel a lot, it's especially important to keep your teaching fresh. Build a niche for yourself and continue to study in it. And take advantage of being in yoga studios to take classes at every destination, and to develop friendships. You may eventually get in the rhythm of visiting the same locations yearly, and this can make the world your yoga home, with friendly colleagues and students to visit at every port.

Constant or even periodic travel can be tough on your relationships and your home life. Your colleagues at your day job, your partner, your children, and your pets will all be affected by your travel schedule. Be sure you have the support network you need before planning an ambitious travel schedule.

DIVERSIFY

Whether you stick close to home or roam, you will need to diversify so that you have income that is not keyed to your being physically present in a classroom. This might mean taking on some administrative work at a studio or for a yoga-related nonprofit. It could mean you spend several hours a week on content creation, making videos or writing useful articles for yoga students, yoga teachers, or both, in a way that you can monetize: charging for video rental, selling ads on a website, writing ebooks, and so on. Maybe you'll develop a parallel expertise in machine Pilates, sewing yoga props, or something that complements your yoga work while expanding your student base and giving you more income potential.

Diversification Plan

Depending on your skill set and your passions, your diversification plan can go in many directions. Take a moment to make notes about what you might do to complement your regular teaching schedule. Then write the first next step to move toward your vision.

YOGA STUDIO OWNERSHIP

If a studio owner is doing their job well, much of their work is invisible. It happens behind the scenes and encompasses a range of tasks from securing and maintaining business licenses and fire inspections to stocking toilet paper. As a teacher, you may see studio owners as swans gliding serenely across the surface of the pond; in reality, they are paddling like heck below the waterline to get where they are going. Because the swans look so peaceful, you may be tempted to dream of opening your own studio.

Articulate Your Vision and Do Your Research

If you do make moves toward studio ownership, go into it with your eyes wide open. Start by writing a business plan. This is a document than can be daunting to draft but that will force you to articulate the vision for your business, to face facts about how the finances will run, to project whether and when it will be profitable. Look at the business plan templates available online at sites like SCORE.org and see if your local chamber of commerce can put you in touch with a business mentor from SCORE or a similar group. (SCORE is a US-based coalition of seasoned businesspeople who volunteer as mentors; you may find a similar outfit if you live outside the United States.) Or look at your local business school to see if the students work with commercial-sector partners on projects like writing a business plan, developing a marketing strategy, or growing a customer base.

Do some research on your own, too. Your local library is a great place to start. The librarians can direct you toward popular, useful business books. Be sure to read Michael Gerber's classic *The E-Myth*, available in a revised edition as *The E-Myth Revisited: Why Most Small Businesses Don't Work and What to Do About It*. The E-Myth is the myth of the entrepreneur: the idea that you can go into business for yourself and do what you love all day long. In reality, as a practitioner, when you open up your own shop, the irony is that you'll have very little time to do what you do best: Practice your craft. Instead, you'll be serving as your own HR department, accounts payable and billable departments, marketing department, facilities and housekeeping departments, and so on, leaving you very little time and energy even to teach yoga, let alone attend to your personal practice.

Marshal Your Resources

Vision alone—even having a beautifully written business plan—is not enough to get you through the creation of a studio. To execute your vision, you need an array of support, from business partners to support services to a supportive spouse and children. You'll want to line all of these up before you even start with staffing or day-to-day operations:

▶ Family and friends for support
▶ Lawyer for incorporation and contracts review
▶ Commercial Realtor to help you find the right space
▶ Accountant to direct you in bookkeeping (or do it) and tax preparation
▶ Banker to help with accounts
▶ Payroll service, or expect to have a lot of contact with your accountant
▶ Software service for the business
▶ Web and graphic designers

Give It Time

Just as it takes at least nine months to see if a class is going to put down firm roots, it takes a long while to see whether a studio will succeed. In your initial business plan, project operational expenses for at least three years, and be sure you have a clear source for the funding. It may take even longer than three years to see a profit. The clearer-eyed you can be at the beginning, the better you'll be able to roll with the punches that small business ownership inevitably throws your way. Expect the unexpected, like a pandemic, and marshal resources and plan ways to adapt. Keep your mission and your goals top of mind, and be sure you give yourself a couple of days off each week and a vacation or two each year.

Carolina Yoga Company

I stumbled into studio ownership. I'd been teaching at Carrboro Yoga from the day Donia Robinson opened it in 2004. On New Year's Day in 2010, I called Donia to see if she'd like to assist me at Kripalu later that month, as she'd done the year before, and she said, "Well . . . I might be moving across the country then. Want to buy a yoga studio?" I did not—but I didn't want the sweet corporate culture to change, as I loved teaching my Monday night yoga for athletes class. My Spinning and yoga student Lies Sapp, a former litigator, had told me she wanted 2010 to be her year of yoga, so when I saw her in class I suggested she might like to buy it. After looking at the books, she said it was profitable but she didn't want a full-time job. However, she was interested in doing half the work for half the profits: Would I join her?

My husband was very much for it from the beginning; I had to think about it. I spent the next morning running a 50-kilometer race, which gave me plenty of alone time to think. By the time I was done, I'd made up my mind. Did I know what I was doing? Not much! But I knew a little, and Lies knew a decent amount about the things that I didn't know, and in the decade since we first started figuring out how to run a studio, we've added two more locations, moved the first one, and expanded our co-ownership to include Hillsborough Spa and Day Retreat and Carolina Massage Institute.

> The biggest takeaway for me: Partner well. Know what you know and what you don't know, and choose strategic partners, either in-house or out of house, to help with the things you don't know.

DEVELOPING CONTINUING EDUCATION AND TEACHER TRAININGS

Training teachers is extremely gratifying work. There is nothing like getting to spend the day in the company of like-minded colleagues to develop a deeper professionalism and expand our tools for serving our students. Leading a room full of teachers in asana practice is a special joy, as we share an understanding of our bodies and a common vocabulary of movement, while at the same time being especially perceptive to subtleties and nuance in sequencing, cueing, and theming.

If you'd like to train teachers, start small by offering short workshops on a topic you've explored in depth. You don't need to know it all; you do need to know something of value and how to convey it. Follow the advice from chapter 10 on developing a workshop. After running several shorter versions of a workshop, you'll be confident and clear on how you can expand it into a full weekend or weeklong training. If you are in the Yoga Alliance network, register as an E-RYT as soon as you can (after one thousand teaching hours and two calendar years past your graduation). This means that other RYTs can count study with you, in workshops or in regular classes, toward their continuing education hours. You can also pay $20 per year to register as a continuing education provider (YACEP), then list your course in the Yoga Alliance's continuing education directory.

In time, you might become involved in a full-featured yoga teacher training. Teacher trainings are a major undertaking. It helps to work inside someone else's to see what parts you would like to handle yourself and where you need support. This might even be enough to convince you that teaching *in* a training is better than constructing one wholesale. If you do choose to create your own, first make sure you are not stepping on any toes locally, especially if you have been teaching inside another program. Your program should be distinct enough that you won't be siphoning off students from a training that has employed you to your mutual benefit. This is good both from a relationship management perspective and for your marketing plan. If you get the all clear, you'll next need to decide whether to affiliate with the Yoga Alliance. If you do, you will design a curriculum that meets their current requirements, detail it on an application, and seek their approval. This may take several rounds of back-and-forth over many months, so do not advertise a start date for your program until it has been cleared.

Whether or not you affiliate your training with the Yoga Alliance, look at their standards and application. This will help you develop policies that will keep you and your trainees clear and safe, including whether, when, and how to give refunds. As you enroll your trainees, be clear on what you want from them. Do you want them to have a particular background? A certain amount of experience as a student? Will you require references? Clear communication with prospective students about the demands of the program, your expectations, and what they can expect as next steps after training will save heartache down the road. Revisit the advice in chapter 2 for those choosing a yoga teacher training, but now envision yourself on the other end of the equation as the trainer, not the trainee. What matters most? How can you attract and enroll those who will ensure the best learning environment for all?

The first round of teacher training will likely be the hardest, as everything will be new to you. Slot in extra care for yourself during YTT weekends or weeks, and make notes after each session about what went well, what didn't, and how you want things to go next time.

When you offer a teacher training, I hope you'll use this book as a manual. It contains everything I tell my teacher trainees, everything I have learned throughout my career, and everything I, as a studio owner, wish teachers knew about how to treat themselves, their clients, their employers, and each other. The more professional each of us strives to be, the healthier the field of teaching yoga and mindful movement will grow. And the healthier the field is, the more people will benefit, teachers and students alike. Thank you for reading, and *namaste*.

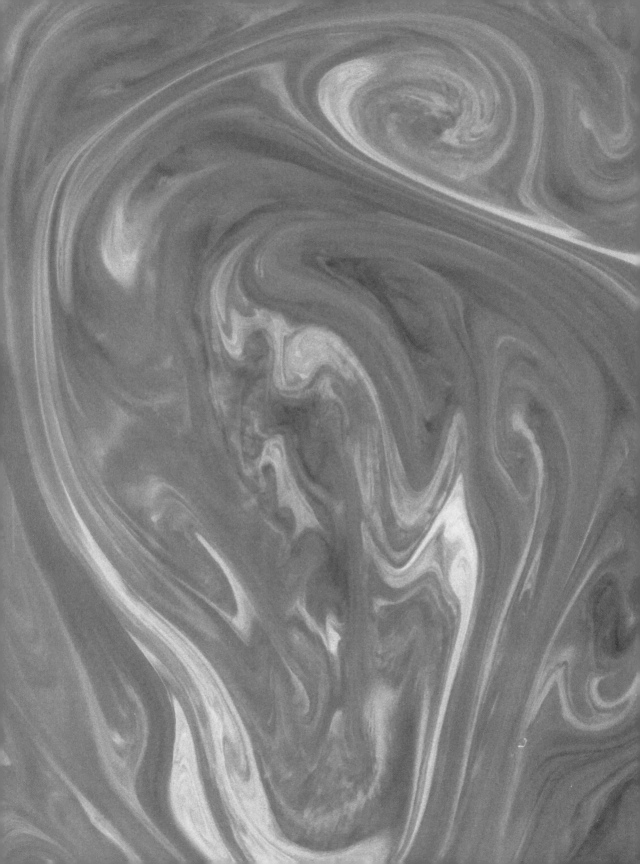

Appendix: A Timeline

· ·

A timeline to keep you on track

Practice yoga
(not necessarily asana).

EVERY DAY

Take a class led by
another teacher,
in person or online.

EVERY WEEK

Put money aside
for taxes.

EVERY PAYCHECK

- ▶ Plan your social media.
- ▶ Update your website.
- ▶ Take a class from
  someone new to you, in
  person or online.
- ▶ Track your expenses
  and reconcile your
  bank accounts.

EVERY MONTH

- ▶ Ask for teaching
  feedback.
- ▶ Plan your newsletter.

EVERY QUARTER

- ▶ Video record your class
  and self-evaluate.
- ▶ Take a workshop.

EVERY SIX MONTHS

▶ Register for a continuing
   education program.

▶ Revisit your goals and
   revise.

▶ Plan a fresh content
   campaign.

▶ Check that your
   financials are in order
   (and file your taxes!).

▶ Renew your insurance.

▶ Update your media kit.

EVERY YEAR

Take fresh photos
and deploy them on
your website, media kit,
and social media profiles.

EVERY OTHER YEAR

▶ Evaluate whether
   Yoga Alliance registry
   is serving you; if so,
   re-up.

▶ Check that your URLs
   are paid up for at least
   three more years.

EVERY THIRD YEAR

Recommended Reading

Brendon Abram, *Teaching Trauma-Sensitive Yoga: A Practical Guide*

David Allen, *Getting Things Done: The Art of Stress-Free Productivity*

Kimberly Carson and Carol Krucoff, *Relax into Yoga for Seniors: A Six-Week Program for Strength, Balance, Flexibility, and Pain Relief*

David Emerson and Elizabeth Hopper, *Overcoming Trauma through Yoga: Reclaiming Your Body*

Donna Farhi, *Teaching Yoga: Exploring the Teacher-Student Relationship*

Michael Gerber, *The E-Myth Revisited: Why Most Small Businesses Don't Work and What to Do About It*

Anna Guest-Jelley, *Curvy Yoga: Love Yourself and Your Body a Little More Each Day*

Leslie Kaminoff and Amy Matthews, *Yoga Anatomy*

Matt Lee and Ted Lee, *Hotbox: Inside Catering, the Food World's Riskiest Business*

Matthew Remski, *Practice and All Is Coming: Abuse, Cult Dynamics, and Healing in Yoga and Beyond*

Erich Schiffmann, *Yoga: The Spirit and Practice of Moving into Stillness*

Jessamyn Stanley, *Every Body Yoga: Let Go of Fear, Get on the Mat, Love Your Body*

Bessel van der Kolk, *The Body Keeps the Score: Brain, Mind, and Body in the Healing of Trauma*

Acknowledgments

· ·

THOUSANDS OF PEOPLE HAVE helped me become a teacher, both directly and indirectly, and I salute them all. To you as a reader, to my yoga teacher trainees, and to every student I've ever had the pleasure of saying *namaste* to: Thank you. You taught me how to do this work. For the masterful dinner party analogy, thank you to Lauren Reese and Tami Roberts of Breathe Yoga Atlanta. Thank you to everyone at the Kripalu Center for Yoga and Health for the decade of support—it is a treat to feel like I have a second yoga home.

Thank you to the women I have had the pleasure of spending my professional hours with: Lies Sapp, Jenni Tarma, Dara Fort, and Alexandra DeSiato. I believe that together, we can do just about anything, from empire building to laughing until we cry—and crying until we laugh.

Thank you to my agent, Linda Konner—a good agent is worth her weight in gold! Thank you to everyone at The Experiment, especially Olivia Peluso for her enthusiasm for this project and the wonderful editing. Olivia, you added immensely to the utility of this book. Thank you.

Thank you to my entire nuclear and extended family for supporting me in this journey. My career is a testament to your help and your faith—especially to the way my husband, Wes, believes in me. Thank you in particular to Martha Harbison, whose multifaceted logistical, financial, emotional, and spiritual support of my career has been one of the greatest gifts of my life. Marty, your investment in my original yoga teacher training has paid huge dividends in helping people through yoga—from my students to their students, to my students' students and beyond. I hope that with this book we have expanded our reach even more in the service of helping people find union and connection.

Index

NOTES

NOTES

NOTES

NOTES

NOTES

About the Author

· ·

SAGE ROUNTREE, PhD, E-RYT 500, moved from a career track in academia to one teaching yoga and training others to do the same, and to do it with clear standards and boundaries to the benefit of their students. Co-owner of the three-studio Carolina Yoga Company in central North Carolina, she directs its teacher trainings, which include both 200-hour and advanced studies offerings that draw students from around the world. Sage has served as a faculty member at the Kripalu Center for Yoga and Health for over a decade, and she has offered workshops and taught at festivals both internationally and around the United States.

Sage's in-person trainings and online courses include lessons in sequencing yoga classes, developing workshops, managing the yoga classroom, and being a professional movement teacher—the subject of this book. A pioneer in yoga for athletes, she has worked with athletes at every level, from youth and amateur athletes to NBA and NFL teams and players. In addition to writing and cowriting nine books, her work has appeared in several publications, and she has been a regular contributor to *Yoga Journal* and *Runner's World*.

Sage lives in Carrboro/Chapel Hill, North Carolina, where she has taught the same regular weekly class for over sixteen years.

sagerountree.com | @sagerountree